Clinical Psychiatry

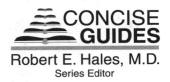

CONCISE GUIDES

Robert E. Hales, M.D.
Series Editor

CONCISE GUIDE TO
Computers in Clinical Psychiatry

Carlyle H. Chan, M.D.

Professor and Vice Chair for Education and Informatics
Department of Psychiatry and Behavioral Medicine
Medical College of Wisconsin
Milwaukee, Wisconsin

John S. Luo, M.D.

Assistant Professor and Director of Psychiatric Informatics
Department of Psychiatry, University of California at Davis
Sacramento, California

Robert S. Kennedy, M.A.

Editor and Program Director
Medscape Psychiatry and Mental Health
and Associate in Psychiatry
Department of Psychiatry and Behavioral Science
Albert Einstein College of Medicine, New York, New York

Washington, DC
London, England

Copyright © 2002 American Psychiatric Publishing, Inc.
ALL RIGHTS RESERVED

Manufactured in the United States of America on acid-free paper
06 05 04 03 02   5 4 3 2 1
First Edition

American Psychiatric Publishing, Inc.
1400 K Street, N.W.
Washington, DC 20005
www.appi.org

Library of Congress Cataloging-in-Publication Data
Chan, Carlyle H.
   Concise guide to computers in clinical psychiatry / Caryle H. Chan,
John S. Luo, Robert S. Kennedy. — 1st ed.
      p. ; cm. — (Concise guides)
Includes bibliographical references and index.
   ISBN 1-58562-100-5 (alk. paper)
   1. Psychiatry—Data processing—Handbooks, manuals, etc.
   [DNLM: 1. Microcomputers—Handbooks. 2. Internet—Handbooks. 3.
Psychology, Clinical—Handbooks. 4. Telemedicine—Handbooks. WM 26.5
C454c 2002] I. Luo, John S., 1966– II. Kennedy, Robert S., 1949– III.
Title. IV. Concise guides (American Psychiatric Publishing)
   RC455.2.D38 C436 2002
   616.89'0025—dc21

                                                    2001058388

British Library Cataloguing in Publication Data
A CIP record is available from the British Library.

CONTENTS

3   Notebook Computers. 17

LIST OF TABLES

7 The Internet

9 Security

LIST OF FIGURES

INTRODUCTION

to the Concise Guides Series

The Concise Guides Series from American Psychiatric Publishing, Inc., provides, in an accessible format, practical information for psychiatrists, psychiatry residents, and medical students working in a variety of treatment settings, such as inpatient psychiatry units, outpatient clinics, consultation-liaison services, and private office settings. The Concise Guides are meant to complement the more detailed information to be found in lengthier psychiatry texts.

The Concise Guides address topics of special concern to psychiatrists in clinical practice. The books in this series contain a detailed table of contents, along with an index, tables, figures, and other charts for easy access. The books are designed to fit into a lab coat pocket or jacket pocket, which makes them a convenient source of information. References have been limited to those most relevant to the material presented.

Robert E. Hales, M.D., M.B.A.
Series Editor, Concise Guides

PREFACE

Futurists Alvin and Heidi Toffler (1995) postulated that the progress of civilization may be considered a series of waves. The first wave was the agricultural revolution, when the switch was made from a nomadic life of hunting and gathering to an agrarian culture, with people living in one location and capable of producing their own food supplies. The second wave was the Industrial Revolution, when people congregated in what are now referred to as urban areas, and factories made it possible to manufacture better goods. The third wave, the current wave, is the information age, in which knowledge and technology have transformed traditional ways of doing just about everything. The hoe, the assembly line, and the computer symbolize these three waves.

In the past several years, the ease with which computers are used has increased tremendously. Gone are the days when it took more than 30 hours to learn a single program. Now, with a graphic user interface, pointing and clicking icons on the screen reduces the learning time for a new program to 2–3 hours. Much of this learning carries over to other new programs; many instructions and commands are standardized. In the science fiction world of *Star Trek,* computers respond to verbal questions and commands. Currently, verbal communication with computers remains much more limited. However, true voice recognition is not that far away.

The personal computer is no longer an isolated device. Through the Internet, a single personal computer can be connected to millions of other computers. The preparation of this book demonstrates, in a very limited way, some of that connectivity. The authors are based in California, Wisconsin, and New York, and chapter revisions crisscrossed the continent several times within the same day via the Internet.

With each chapter revision also came renewed awareness of how this field is constantly and even exponentially changing. Almost daily, new technology is introduced and prices are reduced. Readers should therefore keep in mind that information in a book such as this requires continual updating.

The focus of clinical psychiatry is on taking care of patients. Clinical psychiatrists have new tools to assimilate and manage requisite knowledge, facilitate documentation, and even provide service. On-line Internet learning, electronic record keeping, and telemedicine are just a few examples of the use of computers in clinical care.

In this Concise Guide, we focus on computer applications relevant to the practice of clinical psychiatry, and we provide an introductory reference for clinicians who are either new to computers or contemplating purchasing one for the first time. The chapters may be read independently or sequentially. Chapter 5, "Personal Digital Assistants," is extensive because of the explosion of interest in and applications for these portable computing devices. The glossary is intended to aid readers in navigating the waters of this new area.

We hope that the information presented will have value to the novice computer user. We welcome comments, questions, and suggestions.

Carlyle H. Chan, M.D.
cchan@mail.mcw.edu

John S. Luo, M.D.
jsluo@ucdavis.edu

Robert S. Kennedy, M.A.
Rkennedy@mny.medscapeinc.com

■ **REFERENCE**

Toffler A, Toffler H: Creating a New Civilization: The Politics of the Third Wave. Atlanta, GA, Turner Publishing, 1995

CHOOSING A COMPUTER

Just as there are factors to consider when buying a house or car, there are many questions to ponder when purchasing a computer. Fortunately, the cost of computers has decreased significantly, and computer buyers have a wide selection, whatever their budgets. By answering the following questions, you can help yourself evaluate your needs.

■ SHOULD I UPGRADE MY CURRENT COMPUTER OR BUY A NEW ONE?

When considering whether to upgrade your computer or buy a new computer, ask yourself a few questions. How well is your current computer performing? Is it meeting your current needs? As the saying goes, "If it ain't broke, don't fix it." However, if your programs are running slowly, simply defragmenting the hard drive, adding random access memory (RAM), or replacing your central processing unit (CPU) could speed response significantly. If you are running out of room to store digital photos or other large files, you can either add a hard drive or use another removable storage system. If your pictures and videos are slow to materialize, a new graphics card with more video memory may be all that is required. If your computer does not have the ports you need to connect to new equipment, try to find a card with the needed ports to slip into an expansion slot.

You may reach a point of diminishing returns if you need to upgrade more than a couple of the options mentioned. Also, some older machines are limited to 64 megabytes (MB) of RAM, and in the case of older CPUs, replacing the CPU may mean replacing the entire motherboard. Given the low cost of computers today, it makes sense to look closely at the price differential between upgrading your old computer and purchasing a new one ("Home Computing" 2001). If your computer is more than 2 years old, purchasing a new computer will be less expensive than upgrading.

■ WHEN IS THE BEST TIME TO BUY?

The best time to buy a computer is now. If you wait, there will always be more powerful models and lower prices. However, the longer you wait, the longer you will not be using a computer.

■ WHAT TYPE OF COMPUTER SHOULD I BUY?

The overwhelming majority of desktop computers sold today are IBM-compatible units, made by a variety of manufacturers. Running a distant second are Apple Computer's Macintoshes, or Macs. The latter have a devoted, albeit smaller, following who believe that Macs are superior machines. Because most units sold are IBM-compatible personal computers (PCs), there is significantly more software available for them. Macs have been the computers of choice for students, some researchers, and graphic designers. Because the two systems are not compatible, you must purchase special software that will allow you to change files from one system to another. Although this interchange is possible, translations from one to the other generally are not perfect. PCs and Macs do communicate via the Internet and local area networks (LAN). If you are purchasing a system for home, and IBM-compatible PCs are used at your office, you should probably choose an IBM-compatible PC. Likewise, if your office is Mac based, it will be easier to exchange files with a Mac at home.

■ SHOULD I BUY A DESKTOP, NOTEBOOK, OR HANDHELD COMPUTER?

Like the answer to so many questions, the answer to the question of what type of computer to buy is "it depends." How do you plan to use the computer? What do you plan to use it for? If you do not wish to carry it back and forth between home and office or take it on vacation, and if your family will also make use of it, a desktop model is definitely for you. If you think you will be adding peripheral equipment such as a scanner, surround-sound loudspeakers, or a large monitor, or if your teenager will be using the computer to play video games that require large chunks of video memory, then a desktop is the way to go, although your teenager may well need a separate computer of his or her own. In general, desktop computers are also the least expensive if you decide on a bare-bones model.

If portability is a consideration, then a laptop or notebook computer will be your choice. The power and capacity of notebook computers are rapidly approaching those of desktops. If you must be able to check your electronic mail (e-mail) when you are away from home, having a notebook computer will make this easy. However, if e-mail is the only application you need, consider a BlackBerry Research in Motion (RIM) e-mail device. It is small and gives you instant access to e-mail. The primary disadvantage is the screen size, which makes viewing attachments cumbersome. If you give presentations using computer software, then a notebook computer is a necessity. (Also, see the section regarding presentations in Chapter 5.) If you cannot be without a computer (even when on vacation), choose a notebook.

Handheld computers, or the more commonly used term *personal digital assistants* (PDAs), have not yet replaced notebooks, although that may not be so far away. PDAs have gained in popularity because they are very efficient in what they do. Their initial functions were to keep phone numbers and addresses, schedule appointments, and store to do lists. Now you can purchase a separate keyboard and do word processing, buy a separate modem attachment and surf the World Wide Web wirelessly, or even take digital pictures. Given their small screens and limited editing functions, PDAs perform these new tasks more slowly than the slowest notebooks, yet their ultrasmall size make it possible to carry them in a pocket or purse. At this time, PDAs are noteworthy supplements to portable or desktop computers. (See Chapter 5 for an extensive discussion of PDAs.)

■ HOW MUCH DO I NEED TO SPEND?

There was a period when computers were given away by one's Internet service provider. This seems to have gone the way of the dot-com start-up company. The amount you pay depends on how much you wish to spend and what level of equipment you need. There are three price points: entry level, midlevel, and power user (Table 1–1). More money buys a faster computer with more memory, a larger screen, more peripheral equipment, and more software. Prices have dropped considerably, with entry-level systems starting at $500 and power units starting at about $1,500. It is probably not unreasonable to expect to spend at least $1,000 for a desktop system that does all the things you would like it to do. Prices and equipment can be compared on the Internet at sites such as http://www.cnet.com or http://www.pcmag.com.

Macintosh systems are generally more expensive. iMacs, which are desktop computers, start at around $1,000, and iBooks, which are portables, start at about $1,500. Software is often extra, although it is sometimes bundled with a purchase.

■ WHERE SHOULD I PURCHASE A NEW COMPUTER?

Computers may be purchased from small, independently owned computer stores, mega–computer stores, discount superstores, and even chain discount stores. Computers can also be purchased by mail order and even over the Internet. Specialized computer dealers (both stores and mail-order companies) generally provide better after-sales support than a chain discount store.

Typically, a computer sold by a computer store must be brought back to the store's service center for repair. Some local

TABLE 1–1. Computer systems

Level	Processor speed	Amount of RAM (MB)	Hard drive size (GB)	Monitor size (inches)	Drive	Operating system
Entry level	800 MHz	64	20	15	CD-ROM	Windows 98 or Windows ME
Midlevel	1 GHz	128	30	17	CD-RW	Windows 2000 or XP home
Power user	2 GHz	256	40	19	DVD or CD-RW	Windows XP professional

Note. CD-ROM=compact disc–read-only memory; CD-RW=compact disc–rewritable; DVD=digital video disc; GB=gigabyte; GHz=gigahertz; MB=megabyte; MHz=megahertz; RAM=random access memory.

stores also set up and repair computers at buyers' homes or offices. Find out the warranty and service details before you buy. Mail-order companies have telephone support lines for troubleshooting. (Free telephone support may be time limited.) Many companies will then ship a replacement part, to be installed either by the owner of the computer or by a locally contracted on-site repair service.

Computer and consumer magazines have rated the quality of sales and support services. In general, where you purchase your computer is an issue of cost versus support. Specialty retailers offer more support but have higher prices, whereas chain discount stores may offer better prices but be less helpful.

■ IS THERE A PARTICULAR BRAND I SHOULD BUY?

Deciding on a brand of computer is much like deciding which car you wish to purchase, in that personal preferences are most significant. Design and sticker price may also be considerations. Some vendors design computers more for consumer markets; others design for the business market.

Only a few companies actually manufacture the multiple components inside any computer case. Hence there are only three or four companies that build the CPU chip; a few other companies make floppy disk drives or hard drives. So a computer assembled by a neighborhood computer specialist may have internal components that are similar to those of one made by a well-known manufacturer. Some people purchase computer parts and put together their own computers.

The leading computer makers are Apple, Compaq, Dell, Gateway, Hewlett-Packard, and IBM. Check different periodicals for ratings of computer dependability and service support.

■ ARE THERE OTHER CONSIDERATIONS?

There are other considerations to take into account. Available software could be a significant determinant. If there is software that you need or use and it is written only for a Macintosh, that may be the deciding factor. Some manufacturers bundle different packages of software with their computers. In addition to productivity software (e.g., word processor, database, or spreadsheet software), a games package might be important if you plan to let your children use the computer. If you plan to use digital cameras for video and still photography, a video- and photo-editing package bundled into your purchase could save you a considerable amount of money. However, the type and amount of hardware should be your top priorities when buying a computer.

■ REFERENCE

Home computing: time to upgrade? Consumer Reports, September 2001

2

DESKTOP COMPUTERS

In this chapter, we provide some guidelines and recommendations for buying your first desktop computer or upgrading your current desktop computer. Equipment is constantly changing, and any suggestions given here will be dated by the time of publication. There are many sources of updated recommendations and reviews. Magazines such as *PC Magazine* (http://www.pcmag.com) or *PC World* (http://www.pcworld.com) regularly review software and hardware. In addition, http://www.cnet.com is a Web site dedicated to reviews. In his "Personal Technology" column in the *Wall Street Journal* (http://ptech.wsj.com), Walt Mossberg makes recommendations twice a year.

■ MACINTOSH VERSUS IBM-COMPATIBLE PERSONAL COMPUTER

The first decision is whether to buy a Macintosh (Mac) or an IBM-compatible personal computer (PC). Both types of computers have their advocates and detractors. Apple Computer produces Macs, whereas numerous companies and individuals build and sell IBM-compatible PCs. Macs have been favored by many graphic artists and researchers and have been touted for their stability, multitasking capability, and ease of use. However, although Apple holds about 30% of the precollege market share, its overall computer market share is closer to 3%. The overwhelming majority of desktop computers are IBM-compatible PCs, and significantly more software is therefore available for these computers.

There are only two models of Macintoshes: the iMac and the Power Mac. Versions of each of these models vary in processor speed, memory, drives, and so on. iMacs are less expensive than Power Macs. Motorola makes the PowerPC reduced instruction set computing (RISC) microprocessor chips that drive Macs.

One way to judge which type of computer (Mac or IBM-compatible PC) to buy is to ask yourself, whom do I need to exchange information with, and where can I receive support? If your office or friends have one type of computer, it would be wise to purchase that type, so that you can ask questions and receive help. In the remainder of this chapter, we will focus on IBM-compatible PCs.

■ CONNECTIONS

Many new computers are now legacy free—that is, older-style connections (ports) have been eliminated and newer and faster ports have been substituted. Older ports include parallel ports (typically used for connecting the computer to a printer) and serial ports (used for a mouse, external modem, or other devices). Some of the newer, faster connections include the universal serial bus (USB) and, for video uses, FireWire (Apple) or i-LINK (Sony) IEEE 1394. These new connections transfer data faster and are more stable. Speed is a consideration when large amounts of data, such as scenes from a digital video camera, are being transferred onto a computer. Another advantage of USB connections is that with an external hub, more than one device can be connected through a single port. Computers that are not legacy free typically contain both older and USB ports. If you are upgrading to a legacy-free computer, you might not be able to use your older peripheral equipment (such as a parallel printer) without a new adapter cable.

■ CENTRAL PROCESSING UNIT

The major manufacturer of central processing units (CPUs) or processors for IBM-compatible PCs is Intel, which produces the Pentium and Celeron chips. Advanced Micro Devices (AMD) produces Athlon and Duron chips. Both companies' chips run the same software. The major distinction among chips is speed. Every few months, faster chips are created and sold. Not long ago, chips passed the 1-gigahertz (GHz) speed barrier. Now chips approach and exceed 3 GHz. Few individuals can truly use all this speed. For example, someone who uses a computer for word processing will not see any difference typing on a 400-megahertz (MHz) computer rather than on a 1-GHz computer.

Few new computers today have processors slower than 800 MHz, and you should probably consider that the minimum speed when choosing a new computer. Clinicians who anticipate using speech recognition software may want faster processors, although purchasing more random access memory (RAM) may be more cost efficient. Computers with the newest, fastest processors cost more than those with older, slower processors. One caveat: Chip speed is only one determinant of how fast a computer performs. Factors such as bus speed, L1 and L2 caches, and supporting chip sets also play significant roles.

■ RANDOM ACCESS MEMORY

RAM is the temporary memory that the computer uses, while turned on, to hold the programs and information currently in use. When you turn off the computer, this temporary memory is erased. The CPU can retrieve data from RAM much faster than it can from a hard drive, and thus a computer with a greater amount of RAM runs faster than one with less RAM. Although many computers have 32 or 64 megabytes (MB) of RAM, and older operating systems such as Windows 95 and Windows 98 run fine with this amount of memory, the minimum amount of RAM to be purchased in a new system should be 128 MB. Windows XP requires at least this amount and could probably use more. Memory-intensive programs such as speech recognition software could also use more. Essentially, the more memory you can afford to add, the better your computer will run. RAM chips may be added at a nominal cost and are the best value for speeding up the performance of your software and reducing lock ups and crashes.

■ HARD DRIVE

New programs and new peripheral equipment (e.g., digital cameras, MP3 players) use large amounts of memory, so a hard drive with a minimum of 20 gigabytes (GB) of memory is strongly recommended. If you plan to save digital photo files or MP3 music files frequently, you will need a hard drive with far greater capacity. Also, many new software programs today require several megabytes of hard disk space at installation. The cost of hard drives has decreased considerably in recent years, with prices generally less than $5 per gigabyte. You do have the option of adding either external or internal hard drives later.

■ INPUT/OUTPUT DEVICES OR DISK DRIVES

Most computers still have floppy disk drives, although it is likely that this will not be the case much longer. Floppy disk drives are slow, and floppy disks hold only 1.4 MB of data. The low cost of floppy disks (less than 10¢ each when purchased in volume) led to their widespread use for transferring small files such as written reports. However, they are insufficient for transporting large files such as photos or programs.

Compact disc–read-only memory (CD-ROM) drives are standard equipment in new computer systems. These drives allow you to load new programs onto your computer. CD-ROMs hold 650 MB of data, and the computer can read the information on these discs but not write new information onto them. A new type of drive, the compact disc–rewritable (CD-RW) drive, can both read and write onto rewritable CDs (a compact disc–recordable [CD-R] may be written on once; a CD-RW may be written on multiple times). The ability to copy (burn) information onto a 650-MB CD-ROM may make floppy disks obsolete.

Digital video disc (DVD) drives can show DVD movies while also reading CD-ROMs. DVDs hold more data (4.5 GB) than

CD-ROMs. There are currently three types of recordable DVD drives: DVD-recordable (DVD-R), DVD-rewritable (DVD-RW), and DVD-RAM drives. Information burned by one DVD drive may not be readable by a different company's unit.

Numerous additional informational storage devices exist. Iomega makes Zip drives (which hold 100- and 250-MB cartridges) and Peerless drives (which hold 10- or 20-GB cartridges). Portable storage devices such as Secure Digital, CompactFlash, and Smart-Media permit the transfer of data, including video images and sound files, from one device to another. Streaming tapes, which are not unlike oversized audiocassettes, are used to back up entire hard drives.

■ POINTING DEVICES

The ability to move an on-screen arrow (or cursor) to point at objects and click depends on the use of a mouse, trackball, trackpad, or pointing stick. The older types of mice have a mechanical ball underneath, which rolls as you move the mouse across a flat surface. Newer mice have an optical system that electronically senses the movement. A trackball is essentially a stationary, upside-down mouse. This design allows you to move the ball directly with your fingers. A trackpad is small, flat surface that you touch with your fingers to guide the on-screen cursor or arrow. A pointing stick is a tiny knob, embedded in the center of the keyboard (usually between keys G and H), that is very sensitive to touch. Any directional pressure will cause the cursor to move in that direction. Pointing sticks are mostly found on notebook computers, although a few desktop keyboards have them as well. Which pointing device you choose is a matter of personal preference. Try them all out at a computer store and see what feels best.

■ MONITORS

Cathode-ray tube (CRT) monitors have grown in size and decreased in price. Fifteen-inch monitors are the smallest of these monitors and the least expensive. Seventeen- and 19-inch monitors, which offer greater viewing comfort, are the most popular monitors in terms of size, and their prices are higher. The cost of a 21-inch or larger monitor is typically almost half the cost of a computer system.

The larger the screen, the more desk space the monitor occupies. Liquid crystal display (LCD) monitors (also called flat-panel monitors) are increasing in popularity because they occupy significantly less desk space than CRT monitors and offer comparable image quality. Desktop LCD screens are identical to those of notebook computers. LCD screens are more expensive than CRT monitors, but their cost is decreasing.

■ PRINTERS

It was not too long ago that dot-matrix printers were the norm. Now laser printers and ink-jet printers predominate. Businesses generally use the more expensive laser printers that are built for heavy-duty use, whereas the home consumer usually buys a color ink-jet printer that also prints digital photos. Laser printers are typically more expensive but are becoming more affordable for home use. Ink-jet printers are the least expensive and are quite good for general photo and text printing. The higher-priced printers print faster and with higher resolution.

■ MULTIMEDIA

The CD-ROM drive in your computer will also play audio CDs. Computer speakers with a base amplifier will allow you to hear music while you work on your computer (if what you are doing does not require the CD-ROM drive). The three-dimensional images and sound effects in games and virtual reality function best with their own memory. Sound and multimedia cards are frequently add-on options.

■ SUMMARY

We have described many of the core features to consider when purchasing a computer. Additional devices (peripherals) that can enhance your ability to accomplish tasks are described in Chapter 4.

3

NOTEBOOK COMPUTERS

Personal computers have been around since the 1940s, but it was not until 1975 that one of the first portable computers appeared. That computer, the IBM 5100, had 16–64 kilobytes (KB) of memory (Blinkenlights Archaeological Institute 2001) and cost $9,000–$20,000. Most aficionados of portable computers will acknowledge that the era of portable computing was launched in 1980 with the Osborne 1, a 24-lb. computer (Jones Telecommunications & Multimedia Encyclopedia 2001). Prices at that time were around $2,000 for a portable computer with word processing and spreadsheet capabilities. The first "notebook computer" was the GRiD Compass (Hrothgar's Cool Old Junk Page 2001). It too was produced in 1980, and it weighed 15 lb. Because it used bubble memory, it required an external power source.

Today, notebook computers have significantly more processing power, memory, and disk storage, and their capabilities rival those of desktop computers. Generally, desktop computers will always be 6–12 months ahead of notebook computers in terms of technology because the issues of size, weight, and power consumption must be addressed when dealing with notebooks. Nevertheless, the notebook computer is an indispensable part of computing today. The terms *notebook* and *laptop* are commonly used interchangeably.

■ PURCHASING CONSIDERATIONS

If you are deciding to purchase a notebook computer, you need to consider size, weight, screen size, memory and disk capacity, peripherals, and connectivity. The primary advantage of a notebook computer is portability, but portability can be associated with limitations in form factor (size and shape), capacity, and speed. Notebook computers also typically have smaller screens and are less expandable than desktop computers. If you need to work on files both at home and at the office and you have computers in both places, you might consider simply transferring those files on floppy disks, Zip disks, or recordable compact discs (CD-Rs).

■ USER TYPES

The distinctions between the numerous brands and models of notebook computers, like those of desktop computers, have blurred. There are, however, generalizations based on user type and work type that help determine which notebook is most appropriate. Analyzing the workplace and work type is useful when deciding which notebook features are priorities. Types of notebook users and their needs are described in Table 3–1 and discussed here.

TABLE 3–1.	**User types and their computer uses and requirements**	
User type	**Primary uses of computer**	**Key features required**
Power user	Desktop replacement, statistical analysis	CPU speed, memory, FPU, extensive hard drive space
General user	E-mail, word processing, electronic billing	Comfortable keyboard, large screen
Mobile user	E-mail, word processing, presentations	Less weight; peripherals connected, not integrated
Field user	Word processing, Internet access	Long battery life, wireless capability

Note. CPU=central processing unit; e-mail=electronic mail; FPU=floating-point unit.

Power User

The power user needs all the features of a desktop computer in a mobile package. Raw processing power is needed to run statistical analyses, conduct intense spreadsheet calculations, and handle heavy multitasking. Typically, the power user's notebook computer will have the fastest central processing unit (CPU) with a floating-point unit, the largest amount of memory available, and the fastest and largest hard drive. Most of the peripherals are included, such as a digital video disc (DVD) or compact disc–rewritable (CD-RW) drive, an integrated network interface card (NIC), an integrated modem, and PCMCIA slots. This notebook is essentially a desktop replacement, because the user must have the best resources and peripherals available. The drawbacks are higher cost, more weight, and likely shorter battery life compared with other notebook computers.

General User

The general user demands different capabilities. A large screen is needed for ease of viewing text. Higher resolution and larger font sizes are possible with this larger screen. The general user's notebook computer is primarily used for writing notes, checking schedules, responding to electronic mail (e-mail), and sending bills electronically. Key features include a comfortable keyboard layout and keyboard size. Other peripherals such as a compact disc–read-only memory (CD-ROM) drive, modem, NIC, or floppy disk drive are integrated or connected, depending whether weight or convenience is more important to the user.

Mobile User

The mobile user and the general user have slightly different needs. The mobile user must balance screen size against weight. Currently, notebooks geared toward mobile users typically have smaller liquid crystal display (LCD) panels (approximately 12–13 inches). They weigh 3 lbs. or less and may have special software to prolong battery life. Peripherals such as CD-ROM and floppy disk drives ideally should be available in either a docking or base station; otherwise, they should be connectable via a universal serial bus (USB) or other mechanism. This type of notebook is ideal for a person who uses a computer at the office but frequently travels or gives presentations away from the office. When the notebook is at the office, a full-size keyboard, external mouse, and monitor are connected to the docking station. On the road, the necessary peripherals are brought along and connected when needed.

Field User

The field user demands the ultimate in mobility and battery life. The screen of a field user's notebook is typically smaller and may be specially designed for outdoor use. The processor of choice may be the Transmeta Crusoe, which uses remarkably little power. In a notebook with this processor, the life of one lithium battery may be 7 hours. The field user needs connectivity to the home office. Hence, connections to the Internet are typically wireless, via a specific wireless data network or an adapter connected to a cellular phone. The field user moves extensively—for example, doing consultation-liaison work or visiting multiple clinics or hospitals. Field users may prefer more rugged versions of these notebooks, ones specially built to withstand more wear and tear.

■ COMPONENTS

Notebooks have as many components to consider as desktop computers. Given the demand for small size and low weight, the priorities for notebook components must be assessed as discussed earlier. The following review of the currently available models of each component will assist you in determining whether a particular notebook meets your needs.

Central Processing Unit

The CPU is the brain of the computer, responsible for processing software commands and information. There are many different manufacturers of CPUs, but it is advisable to purchase a notebook with an Intel, Advanced Micro Devices (AMD), or Transmeta CPU. The processing power of the CPU is often confused with its clock speed (measured in megahertz [mhz] and gigahertz [ghz]). CPU performance is also determined by the internal architecture of each CPU and how that architecture governs communication with other parts of the computer system. Hence, different model 800 mhz CPUs may still exhibit marked differences in how quickly they perform certain tasks. Notebook CPUs are designed to use less energy and dissipate less heat. Beware of a notebook computer with a price much lower than that of other computer manufacturers. Some manufacturers use desktop CPUs in their notebooks. Although functionally such a CPU has the same speed, it will not have the lower power consumption and low heat generation. Heat is the enemy of the notebook computer because in small quarters, heat is more likely to ruin delicate transistor circuitry.

Memory

Purchase as much memory as you can afford. If cost is a factor, then determining the proper CPU for your needs becomes a priority; memory can always be added later, usually at a lower price.

Video Chip Set

The video chip set of the notebook computer determines resolution. A better-quality video chip set is usually not crucial, unless high resolutions and greater amounts of color are needed (e.g., to adequately display magnetic resonance images or single photon emission computed tomography scans). Checking the video chip set is important when determining whether the notebook will support the external monitor that may be used when the computer is docked. Some video chip sets of notebook computers are capable of generating television output, which means that a television may be used in lieu of an external monitor. This feature is useful because of the frequent problems of compatibility between LCD projectors and notebook computers. Finally, more video memory is needed if the notebook is to be used to handle high inputs such as video signals.

PC Card

Most notebook computers come with PC Card slots, also called PCMCIA slots. These business card–sized slots accept components such as NICs, modems, FireWire cards, and connections to floppy disk and CD-ROM drives. These slots are found in nearly all notebook computers and are essential for adding components. Having fewer integrated peripherals means less weight and longer battery life, although at the cost of function. The PC Card slot permits the addition of desired features when needed.

Pointing Device

On a notebook, the integrated pointing device is typically a trackball, a trackpad, or a pointing stick in the keyboard. (See Chapter 2 for descriptions of these devices.) The choice of pointing device is a matter of personal preference, but there are a few factors to consider. The trackball is best suited for those who have used one with a desktop computer. This device may be located in an area below the main keyboard or as an attachment to the side. The trackpad is located in the area below the main keyboard and is the most common of all integrated pointing devices. The primary disadvantage is that to use it, you must move your hand off the keyboard, which decreases typing speed. The pointing stick is found on only a few models of notebook computers. Its location in the middle of the keyboard allows for a briefer interruption of typing. However, many users find the pointing stick difficult to use.

Modem

The modem may be integrated or be added via the PC Card slot. Windows operating system modems and integrated modems are called softmodems or software-based modems. These modems do not have a chip with built-in modem functions; instead, they have a combination of a digital signal processing chip and software that emulates the modem functions. The advantage of this type of modem is that it is easily updated. However, if you choose to use alternative operating systems such as Linux or BeOS, this type of modem is usually not supported.

Network Interface Card

The NIC is now often integrated in the notebook, making an additional PC Card NIC unnecessary. However, if this card is built into the motherboard, it is not upgradable and it will drain battery power. The NIC is necessary to access local area networks (LANs) and is useful for transferring files directly from the notebook to another computer via a peer-to-peer network connection.

Parallel Port

The parallel port is a standard feature of most notebooks. Although it is largely ignored, it serves a variety of functions. It is the standard mechanism for connecting notebook computers to printers. It is also used for several other peripherals. For example, an Iomega Zip drive, CD burner, or external hard drive may be connected via the parallel port. Software such as LapLink still uses the parallel port as one mechanism to connect computers when a peer-to-peer network cannot be set up.

Serial Port

Like the parallel port, the serial port is a notebook standard. This port is used for an older popular personal digital assistant (PDA) to connect to the main computer. Many older peripherals such as external modems and serial-port mice connect using this port. Today, the USB port has supplanted the serial port.

Universal Serial Bus Port

The USB port has largely replaced the serial port. This port allows for higher transmission speeds as well as management of several devices simultaneously. In addition, peripherals may draw power off the USB port for small devices such as a notebook light. In newer operating systems using the USB port, peripheral devices can be switched without the need for shutting down the computer (this is called hot swapping). The USB port allows for fewer interrupt requests (IRQs) to be devoted to peripherals. An IRQ is essentially a channel of communication to the CPU. When the mouse is moved, it sends a signal to the CPU via the IRQ. With this signal, the CPU knows to interrupt its activity and decide what to do next. Thus, fewer interrupts translates to a faster system.

Infrared Port

The infrared port is a typical feature of most notebook computers. It allows for cableless connections to printers. Users of PDAs can also use the infrared port to synchronize without cables. This port has not been widely used, because transmission speed is slower than with cables and because the signal strength is not very strong, making it necessary to keep the infrared device close to the computer. Ambient light may also interfere with the signal. Finally, the devices must remain within the line of sight of each other for the infrared transmission to work.

CD-ROM Drive

The CD-ROM drive is an essential drive because most software programs are now sold on CD-ROMs. Before CD-R and CD-RW drives were available for notebooks, other storage mechanisms such as Iomega Zip drives were popular for storage and transfer of large files or large numbers of files. The CD-ROM is a popular medium for all computers and is quite cost-efficient. Now, a CD-R or CD-RW drive is a popular option for users with files larger than 1.44 megabytes (MB) (the maximum storage space on a 3.5-inch floppy disk).

Floppy Disk Drive

The floppy disk drive is still a peripheral in most computers. It is largely a legacy device, given the relative infrequency that software is sold on floppy disks. However, because so many computers have floppy disk drives, and because floppy disks are so inexpensive (less than 10¢ each when bought in bulk), the floppy disk continues to be used for exchanging small files.

Alternative Drives

A number of replacements for standard floppy disk drives exist for notebook computers, including the SuperDrive, the Zip drive, and the 2.88-MB floppy disk drive. Using these devices is faster and cheaper than using 3.5-inch floppy disks. They are useful only if you do not intend to share files with users of other computers, or if you intend to share files with users of computers with the same types of drives.

Docking Station and Port Replicator

The docking station and the port replicator permit the connection of a notebook computer to one device, which in turn is connected to many other peripherals. A docking station is a frame with connections that enable the notebook computer to function like a desktop computer. A port replicator duplicates the serial, USB, parallel, and external monitor ports and expands the number of ports. A full-size keyboard and a large external monitor can attach via the docking station or port replicator to a notebook with a small screen and/or a small keyboard, making the system more comfortable for prolonged use at home or at the office. Most manufacturers of notebook computers have their own port replicators that connect to the notebook via a proprietary port. General replicators for any notebook are available that connect via a USB or PC Card.

802.11b or Wi-Fi

A wireless LAN access card is the latest integrated device in notebook computers. This device allows for wireless connection to LANs and often the Internet. 802.11b is the wireless LAN standard protocol. This protocol makes it possible for one manufacturer's wireless device to communicate with another manufacturer's device. Wi-Fi is a further certification that guarantees interoperability. For the user who often travels in a general area around the access point, this device may be extremely convenient. For general use such as browsing, the transfer rate of 11 megabits per second (Mbps) is adequate. However, for large file transfers, this rate may be a bit slow. When this device is used, the LAN is also exposed to hackers. Only 33% of wireless LANs have appropriate security protocols in place and have dynamic Internet Protocol (IP) address designation (an automatic network connection process) (Ellison 2001). If you do not take these precautions, unscrupulous users can gain access to your Internet connection and to your data on the LAN.

■ SECURITY MEASURES

The notebook computer is an easy target for theft, and notebook users must take precautions. Security measures are described here (and discussed more fully in Chapter 9).

Physical Security

Modern notebook computers have a mount where a cable can be secured to the notebook. This mount is now an industry standard. The cable is then wrapped and locked to a stationary device.

Motion Sensor

Port Inc. has developed a device that is motion sensitive. The device generates a very loud sound designed to draw attention as well as produce discomfort.

Tracking

Computrace is a software client that lies dormant in the notebook computer. If the notebook is stolen, the next time that it is connected to either the Internet or a telephone line, it will dial back to the manufacturer and provide the telephone number or IP address.

Encryption

One mechanism to keep sensitive information from exposure is encryption. It may not be convenient or speed efficient to have the entire hard drive encrypted. However, if all data are located in one directory for backup purposes, this same directory can be kept encrypted.

Viewing

Notebooks as well as desktops can be viewed at many angles. If you wish to prevent your neighbor from viewing your screen, buy a special screen overlay that permits only direct viewing. This capability will soon be incorporated into the LCD panel itself.

■ PURCHASING A NOTEBOOK

As is true of desktop computers, notebook computers can be purchased at a variety of places. In most cases, there are home and corporate product lines. The higher-end notebook computers are often not available for viewing in retail stores. However, you can examine and test the keyboards and screens of lower-priced models.

Keep in mind that a notebook will likely not be very upgradable. You can increase memory and hard disk space easily, but changing the motherboard and CPU are not as simple as with desktop computers. In addition, the other chip sets (e.g., the modem, the integrated NIC, and the video card) are typically soldered into the motherboard. Your notebook should give you approximately 2 years of use with minor upgrades. When further upgrades are needed, it makes more financial sense to buy a new system.

■ REFERENCES

Blinkenlights Archaeological Institute: Pop quiz: what was the first personal computer? Available at: http://www.blinkenlights.com/pc.shtml. Accessed December 14, 2001

Ellison C: Exploiting and protecting 802.11b wireless networks. Extreme-Tech, September 4, 2001 (serial online). Available at: http://www.extremetech.com/article/0,3396,s%253D1024%2526a%253D13880,00.asp. Accessed December 14, 2001

Hrothgar's Cool Old Junk Page. GRiD Compass 1101. Available at: http://www.total.net/~hrothgar/museum/Compass/index.html. Accessed December 14, 2001

Jones Telecommunications & Multimedia Encyclopedia: Osborne Computer Corporation. Available at: http://www.digitalcentury.com/encyclo/update/osborne.html Accessed December 14, 2001

4

PERIPHERAL EQUIPMENT

One way to expand computers beyond their physical size and capabilities is to add on or connect peripherals.

■ SCANNERS

Scanners are devices that "read" paper copies of text or graphics and transform them into digital information that the computer can understand and manipulate. For example, if you wish to put a typed page into your personal computer (PC), you can use a scanner to read the page into the PC. The page enters the computer as a graphic image or picture, just as a fax is a picture of a page. A specialized software program does the job of reading or scanning the page image and attempts to "recognize" the words on the page (this process is called optical character recognition). It then converts the page image into an ASCII format for word processing or text editing. It marks all the words that it was not able to determine.

Scanners are popular and inexpensive and have become quite sophisticated in terms of the quality of images that they can capture. There are even special scanners just for business cards. For the average consumer, scanner choice should be based on features and price, because quality is comparable.

Other specialized scanners can be used for educational or business purposes. Bar code scanners read standard bar codes and generally come with software that inputs the codes into a database. These scanners are useful in clinics and in other situations in which speedy access and confidentiality are important. (See the section "Palm OS PDAs" in Chapter 5 for examples.)

Optical mark scanners read test and survey results. They read the pencil dots that are marked on a form. The placement of the dots is interpreted, and they are converted into test scores or survey results by means of specialized software (e.g., Teleforms). These scanners are very expensive and are considered single-purpose scanners.

Scanners make getting data into a computer easier. Scanning saves the user the time it would take to enter the information manually.

Scanners come with scanning and editing software and often optical character recognition software. Learning to use the scanning software and the optical character recognition software and making preliminary adjustments (e.g., adjustments of brightness and color intensity) should take approximately 30–45 minutes.

■ DIGITAL CAMERAS (STILL PHOTOGRAPHY)

Digital cameras have changed the landscape of photography. Images are stored on memory modules or memory cards instead of on film. The images are then transferred to a PC via a cable. The memory in the camera can then be erased so that you can take more pictures. The quality of the picture depends on the quality of the lens and the charge-coupled device. Cameras are rated on the basis of the megapixel capacity of the charge-coupled device. Many models are available, from inexpensive and uncomplicated models to very expensive and sophisticated models.

Resolution of a picture can also depend on the amount of storage in the camera. A memory card can store many low-resolution pictures, like those needed for the World Wide Web or for typical home viewing. High-quality photographs require many megabytes (MB) of storage, and most cameras offer the choice between low- and high-resolution photographs. Swapping memory cards is another option of many digital cameras. Instead of returning to the computer to transfer the pictures when the card is filled, you can insert another blank card and continue taking photographs.

You should read some of the manual that comes with the camera, familiarize yourself with the buttons, and learn how to transfer images to your PC. Gaining a basic understanding takes approximately 10–15 minutes. Learning about the sophisticated features requires more time.

■ DIGITAL VIDEO CAMERAS

Digital video cameras have added the dimension of digital photography to moving pictures. The quality is superior, and still photographs can be used from a single frame of digital video. Video can be recorded to digital tapes that you insert into the camera. Alternatively, many computers offer high-speed connections that allow you to plug the camera directly into the computer and record video directly onto the computer's hard drive. These digital video cameras are somewhat expensive.

Smaller digital video cameras, also known as webcams, have become quite popular. These are, essentially, video lenses that connect to the computer only. They can be used to record still images or video directly onto the computer or to connect, over the Internet, people with similar cameras. These small cameras are made to sit on top of the computer monitor and can be used for videoconferencing as well, although their image quality does not make them ideal for this. They vary in price, from inexpensive to expensive, depending on quality.

Many of these cameras come with software that allows rudimentary manipulation of images and some crude video editing. You can buy more sophisticated video-editing software that has many professional editing capabilities.

Many webcams come with some simple videoconferencing software or take advantage of the conferencing capabilities of the computer's operating system. This type of software can be used for basic videoconferencing over the Web.

Read some of the manual, become familiar with the buttons of the camera, and find out how to transfer images to your computer. Expect to spend approximately 10–15 minutes learning about the camera after you have loaded the software. Understanding the sophisticated features takes longer.

■ MULTIFUNCTION OR ALL-IN-ONE UNITS

One popular office peripheral is the all-in-one unit. Rather than buying a scanner, a fax machine, a printer, and a copier, you can purchase an all-in-one unit with all these capabilities. Both ink-jet and laser models are available. The quality is quite good. The only drawback of an all-in-one unit is that if one component does not function properly, you lose all four capabilities while the unit is being repaired.

Multifunction units are moderately easy to use. Setup takes 45 minutes to 1 hour and generally involves attachment to a computer.

■ SPEECH RECOGNITION TECHNOLOGY

For decades, people have wished for machines that could accept voice input. Speech recognition technology was demonstrated at the 1939–1940 New York World's Fair, but since then progress has been slow. Adequate hardware and sophisticated software were necessary.

In PCs, speech recognition technology primarily involves software, but hardware that can handle the necessary processing power is also needed. Speech recognition software requires a sufficiently fast central processing unit (CPU) (newer chips rather than older ones), preferably at least 128 MB of random access memory (RAM), a sound card, and a headset with a microphone that has noise-canceling capability. (For a discussion of speech recognition software, see Chapter 6.)

Installation is fairly simple, but the major manufacturers of speech recognition software differ with regard to training. Some software involves only 5 minutes of training; with other software, training takes 10–15 minutes. The person being trained reads a number of preselected paragraphs aloud. Overall setup generally takes 30 minutes or more.

■ PERMANENT STORAGE

Permanent storage refers to devices that store your programs and information while you are working on the computer and keep all your data while the computer is off. Floppy disks and hard drives (also referred to as hard disks) store data and programs. A hard disk is generally located inside the computer box, whereas the other types of storage are mostly removable. Data can be stored on a compact disc–read-only memory (CD-ROM) or a Zip disk or with tape backup devices. Software programs are sold on floppy disks or CD-ROMs.

One standard page of typed text, with no formatting, requires between 1.5 and 2 kilobytes (KB) of memory. The same page with different typefaces and type sizes could occupy 10 KB of memory. The same page with graphics could take 200 KB. A detailed one-page picture or photograph (uncompressed) may occupy 2 MB or more of disk space. *Encyclopædia Britannica* takes up

- 225,000 pages
- 33 volumes
- 300 1.44-MB (3.5-inch) floppy disks
- one 500-MB hard disk
- one 680-MB CD-ROM

Zip disks are essentially large-capacity (100- and 250-MB) floppy disks. They used to be fairly popular, but they have given way to CD-ROMs (650-MB capacity) as CD-ROMs and CD-ROM burners have come down in price. A new removable disk drive from Iomega called the Peerless drive uses FireWire or universal serial bus (USB) connections and takes 10- and 20-gigabyte (GB) disks.

Memory cards are small removable cards that can be used in the PCMCIA (or PC Card) slot of your portable computer or digital camera. When the memory card is full, you can replace it with another. A card reader can be attached to your computer for opening and saving files. The most common types of memory cards are CompactFlash, SmartMedia, and Memory Stick. You must use the right type of card for your digital camera or computer. Memory cards are available in various densities, as are other storage devices.

■ PROJECTORS

Computer projection devices use either liquid crystal display (LCD) or Digital Light Processing (DLP). In an LCD projector, images come from three LCD chips. In a DLP unit, a small chip covered with tiny mirrors deflects light toward or away from system optics to create an image on the screen. With the advent of DLP, black and white definition improved, and units were made lighter.

Brightness is a critical factor in projectors. The level of brightness should be approximately 800–1,200 lumens for normal indoor light. Some units exceed 3,000 lumens. A second factor is resolution. Higher-resolution, eXtended Graphics Array (XGA; 1024 × 768 pixels) projectors generally cost more than lower-resolution, Super Video Graphics Array (SVGA; 800 × 600 pixels) projectors. Finally, weight is a consideration if you plan to carry your projector with you. New units now weigh as little as 3 lb.

Brighter is better, and often the more expensive units offer greater brightness as well as other features such as sound, a variety of inputs, less weight, and smaller size. Smaller units often have small speakers; an external loudspeaker will be needed if better sound is required.

Projectors are quite expensive. As they become more popular, prices will drop, but the better units have not gone much under $2,000 for years. Many projectors cost between $3,000 and $4,000.

■ SURGE PROTECTORS

Surge protectors are an important component of any computer system. A surge protector is a power strip with one or more plugs, into which you plug your computer, monitor, scanner, and any other peripherals with power plugs. These devices protect your valuable electronic components against electrical surges, which are quite common and may damage sensitive electronic equipment. Electric-line noise, a common source of minor surges, can come from other activated electrical equipment (e.g., power saws, copiers, laser printers, even equipment on another floor or in another building).

Less expensive surge protectors clamp voltage when they sense that a 300- to 400-volt surge is coming through the electric lines. These surge protectors protect equipment against catastrophic damage but do not stop some of the low-level noise or surges that occur. The better surge protectors block surges entirely. As a rule, more expensive surge suppressors work better, and less expensive units become ineffective over time.

■ UNINTERRUPTIBLE POWER SUPPLY

Uninterruptible power supplies (UPSs) are electronic devices that constantly watch the power coming into your computer. If the UPS senses (within milliseconds) that there is a decrease in power or even a reduction in electricity that would interrupt your computer's power supply, it activates a battery and keeps your computer running without interruption or harm. UPSs are fairly inexpensive. If you live in an area where power brownouts, power drops, or blackouts occur frequently, you should seriously consider buying a UPS. If the device prevents your computer from turning off and saves your data even once, it is worth the cost. UPSs also have built-in surge protectors to protect your computer against surges and spikes. Typically a UPS unit provides only a few minutes of supplemental power, but this should be enough time for you to save what you are currently working on and then shut down your computer.

■ LOUDSPEAKERS

Speakers are usually bundled with a computer system, although low-end or business systems may not have them. They require a sound card. Some speakers are incorporated into the monitor but are less than adequate for music. Reasonable-quality sound may be obtained with a pair of external speakers supplemented with a separate base subwoofer. Many sound systems can be purchased for well under $100.

■ SUMMARY

Peripherals add more features or capacity to your computer. You should consider spending more for higher-quality peripherals or more features. As you upgrade your computer, some peripherals will remain useful, but others may need to be upgraded as well.

5

PERSONAL DIGITAL ASSISTANTS

Personal digital assistants (PDAs) have quickly emerged as essential tools in the practice of medicine. New software is released daily, and newer devices are developed and available almost monthly. An Internet search using the keyword *personal digital assistant* or *PalmPilot* yields thousands of Web sites. It is difficult to catalog all the available software and hardware extensively, but this Concise Guide serves as an entry into the world of portable computing.

The terms *personal digital assistant, handheld computer,* and *PalmPilot* are often used interchangeably. Palm is a brand name, and PalmPilot is an outdated model. The term *handheld computers* has been more closely identified with Windows CE units because of their close association with the other Windows operating systems (OSs). However, we use the term *personal digital assistant* in a generic sense, encompassing the term *handheld computer*.

■ REASONS FOR BUYING A PDA

PDAs are not replacements for notebook computers. Why then should you purchase such a device? One way to answer that question is to analyze your practice patterns and information needs. If you work primarily in one office and handle few calls away from the office, a PDA or notebook computer may be unnecessary. However, if you work on a consultation-liaison service and must move often and quickly from one location to the next, a PDA, which fits into a pocket or purse and is thus more portable than a notebook, would be useful to you. Users who switch locations less frequently (e.g., daily) will likely find a notebook computer more amenable to their computing needs.

Another perspective is that a PDA is not a replacement for a desktop or notebook computer but is a valuable extension. If you have a PDA, you will have quick access to information with minimal or no startup time. In addition, much of the information stored on your PDA is also accessible on your desktop or notebook computer. In this process, called synchronization, information is copied from your PDA onto your desktop or notebook computer and vice versa. A change in appointments made on your PDA will be reflected on your notebook's or desktop's personal information manager after synchronizing. Similarly, if you keep track of appointments on your notebook or desktop computer, synchronization will permit you to view your schedule on your PDA. The desktop or notebook serves as backup for the PDA as well as an alternative means of entering and looking up information.

■ HISTORY

The inspiration for PDAs dates back to the early 1990s. Electronic organizers became portable telephone and address books with some calendar and appointment functions. These devices had tiny keyboards for data entry and no connection to desktop computers. Subsequently, an early PDA, Apple Newton, permitted entry via handwriting recognition and had no optional keyboard available.

By the mid-1990s, the concept of palmtop computing was born, with the emphasis on small size, ease, and speed and with the acknowledgment that users wanted a device that was instantly on and ready to work—PalmPilot. Palm, maker of PalmPilot, also added interfacing: the device and the desktop computer would exchange information (addresses, appointments, electronic mail [e-mail]) regularly. These devices were based on Palm OS. From then on, a pen or stylus became the primary means for interacting with the device.

After the success of PalmPilot, competing devices were produced that were based on Microsoft's Windows CE, developed specifically for these handheld devices. Pocket PC 2002 is the most recent reiteration of Windows CE.

■ PDA OPTIONS

A myriad of devices fit into the PDA category. Each device may have its own advantage and focus. We will discuss devices that not only offer the electronic date book, address book, memo pad, and to do list features but have medical applications as well.

PDAs are categorized by OS. Today, two OSs—Palm OS and Pocket PC—dominate the PDA market. Pocket PC is essentially Windows CE with a few improvements. EPOC, which has a strong following in Europe, is a distant third. Linux has found its way onto PDAs, either as the native OS or as a replacement for the existing OS. There are many other devices with their own proprietary OSs, but these devices have limited applicability in the medical arena.

In general, handheld computers are slightly larger than PDAs. Handhelds typically include a small, integrated keyboard with a larger screen. The majority of handheld computers use Windows CE. These units are between notebook computers and PDAs in terms of function and capacity.

■ CHOOSING A PDA

Deciding which PDA to purchase is akin to deciding whether to purchase an IBM-compatible personal computer (PC) or a Macintosh (Mac). Although EPOC PDAs are very good, they have only a small percentage of market share and an uncertain future. Unless you know many other people who are using EPOC PDAs, your best bet is to decide between Palm OS and Pocket PC PDAs. Linux PDAs are primarily for users who are already using Linux on their desktop or notebook computers and who can write their own programs to fit their needs. Deciding which OS to use largely hinges on which OS and device have the best features for your information needs. To determine which system fits your needs best, consider the differences noted in Table 5–1.

TABLE 5–1.	Features of Palm operating system and Pocket PC personal digital assistants	
Feature	**Palm OS PDA**	**Pocket PC PDA**
Multimedia (video, audio)	++	+++++
Microsoft Office integration	+++	+++++
Battery life	+++++	++
Personal information manager transfer of information	++++	++
Medical software	+++++	+++
Web browsing	+++	++++

Note. OS=operating system; PDA=personal digital assistant.

Palm OS PDAs

Palm OS currently leads the PDA market, with numerous companies licensing the OS for use in their devices. Palm OS PDAs have longer battery lives than do Pocket PCs and are on nearly instantly. More important, a large developer base is associated with Palm OS PDAs. Deciding which Palm OS device to use is complicated. There are many features to consider, and some of the differences are subtle. If possible, ask people who use Palm OS PDAs what they have found to be the advantages and disadvantages. The main differences concern memory expansion, form factor (size and shape), peripherals (attachments), screen resolution, and battery type. As your computing needs change and new options appear, your PDA selection will also change.

The Palm (http://www.palm.com) product line of PDAs has been around for many product generations. The primary advantage of buying a Palm OS PDA is that the OS is upgradable, because it resides in flash memory. Data in flash memory can be replaced but are maintained unless power is lost. In addition, many peripherals (e.g., keyboards, styli, modems, backup modules, and wireless network adapters) fit this platform. Palm has switched the serial/universal service bus (USB) adapter with each product line but intends to standardize the adapter in future products. In general, PDAs have the standard 160 × 160 pixel screens. New Palm models accommodate Secure Digital (SD) cards and MultiMediaCards (MMCs), permitting memory expansion.

The Handspring (http://www.handspring.com) product line has been a great success, in large part because of the Springboard module. Modeled after Nintendo GameBoys, this expansion slot serves as a docking port for other hardware peripherals. Modules available include modems, extra memory, keyboards, presentation modules, backup modules, global positioning system (GPS) units, MP3 players, wireless local area networks (LANs) adaptors, cellular telephones, and game ports. Handspring's competitive advantage is that a wide variety of peripherals are available, and multiple vendors make those modules. These peripherals are proprietary and cannot be used with non-Handspring devices. In addition, Handspring has chosen to modify Palm OS for its PDAs, and because the OS resides in read-only memory (ROM), it cannot be upgraded.

HandEra (http://www.handera.com), formerly known as TRG Products, produces one of the more popular Palm OS PDAs in the medical field. This popularity is due mainly to the fact that HandEra was the first developer to add significantly more memory, through inclusion of a CompactFlash (CF) card slot. CF cards are one of the few industry standards (they are also used in digital cameras), and additional memory is available in up to 128-megabyte (MB) sizes. In the newer HandEra 330 model, the Graffiti input area is virtually displayed, resulting in a larger viewing area. In addition, landscape mode rotates the screen sideways, permitting you to see more columns in a spreadsheet, for example. The HandEra 330 handles both a CF card and an SD card and has three power-supply options. The OS in both the HandEra 330 and the TRG Pro can be upgraded.

Sony (http://www.sony.com) is new to the Palm OS PDA market, and there are several compelling reasons to purchase these devices. Memory Sticks used in Sony PDAs and other Sony products (e.g., notebook computers, desktop computers, digital cameras) are interchangeable. Memory Sticks come in 8-, 16-, 32-, 64-, and 128-MB sizes. Sony PDAs have Jog Dials. A Jog Dial is a wheel used with one hand to switch between applications or to scroll in certain software programs. It has not been well received, but it is certainly a matter of preference. For synchronization, all Sony PDAs use the USB port, which is faster than the serial port. Sony offers the highest screen resolution; two models have 320×320 pixel resolution. This higher resolution is better for showing color digital pictures or viewing small video clips.

Symbol Technologies (http://www.symbol.com) makes several Palm OS PDAs with built-in bar code scanners, which permit utilization of information encoded in bar codes. One hospital uses the scanner to double-check patients before administering medications. Another potential use is to simplify management of drug sample inventories. Symbol devices are slightly larger than most PDAs and are built to withstand temperature extremes and 4-foot drops. Symbol is one of the only companies to build both Palm OS and Windows CE machines.

Cellular telephone–Palm OS PDA hybrids also exist. Samsung, Kyocera International, and Handspring offer these hybrids. The advantage of these devices is that they integrate the PDA address book with the cellular telephone dialing function. One disadvantage is the limited expansion capability. A different way to add PDA-stored telephone numbers to the cellular telephone memory is to use a service of fusionOne (http://www.fusionone.com). This company offers software that allows the user to designate the telephone numbers stored in the PDA that should be added to the cellular telephone memory. The user marks the numbers with an exclamation point. After synchronization with an Internet connection to the fusionOne server, the telephone numbers are sent via Short Message Service (SMS) to be stored in the user's Palm OS PDA. Also, several vendors sell programs that upload the telephone numbers.

Basic Functions

The Palm OS PDA has several standard features. Most are self-explanatory with experimentation and are well covered in the user manual. Those functions are not discussed here. Instead, we will focus on lesser-known tips and tricks.

Repeated pressing of any of the four buttons at the bottom of the PDA will result in the cycling of the different categories of each button (i.e., date book, address book, to do list, and memo pad). There is also a shortcut to cutting and pasting entries: Highlight the item you wish to copy by dragging your stylus across it, make a diagonal upstroke from lower left to upper right, write the letter *c* (for *copy*), move to where you wish to paste the copied item, repeat the diagonal upstroke, and write the letter *p* (for *paste*).

Calculator.   The calculator button can be remapped to other software if it is not used often. (Tap Preferences and then Button.)

Find.   The built-in Find feature searches only the date book, address book, to do list, and memo pad in the PDA. To search information in other software, you must use FindHack (see the section entitled "HackMaster," later in this chapter).

Date Book.   You may quickly access notes by tapping on the note icon in the day view.

Address Book.   Choose one entry as your business card. While in the editing window, tap the menu button and then tap Set Business Card. If you tap Yes, that entry will then have a Rolodex-type icon attached, signifying that this is your business card. To beam your business card quickly to other PDAs, hold the address book button for 2 seconds. The card will be transmitted without being selected.

To Do List.   To better organize your to do list, you may modify or add new categories.

Memo Pad.   The memo pad has a limited file space of 4 kilobytes (KB), or about two pages of typed text.

HotSync.   Most users will not have to modify this task. It may be activated by pressing the HotSync button on the cradle or on the PDA applications screen. If you tap Menu, you will find a series of options. Except for Connection Setup, the majority of them will not be used by most people. Tap Connection Setup, then Edit, and then Details, where you will find the connection speed. On the desktop, right click on the HotSync icon and then select Menu, where you will set the connection speed. Connection speed set on your desktop computer and the PDA must match; otherwise, connection will not be possible.

Security.   Many users do not set security passwords. If confidential information is kept in your PDA, you should consider using this feature. This mechanism hides all your records, necessitates the use of a password when you open the device, and establishes password block to accessing information on Palm Desktop. Although this security is minimal, it is better than leaving your valuable information exposed.

Preferences.   Most of these settings are self-explanatory, but here are some tips. Tap Buttons and select Pen. Now the upstroke key can be set to Beam Data. This feature is extremely useful. Normally, when beaming an entry such as an address, you must tap the entry to highlight it, then tap Menu, and then select Beam address. With this upstroke feature, after the item is selected, an upstroke will then beam the item, saving one motion. If you do not change this preference, an upstroke activates a screen that shows how to form the various letters, numbers, and symbols of the Graffiti alphabet.

When the screen is not responsive, try selecting Digitizer, which resets the way in which the screen is mapped.

The General selection leads to Beam Receive. Turning Beam Receive off will prolong battery life because the PDA will not waste energy checking the infrared port. There is a shortcut that allows you to turn on the infrared port for one input beam without resetting Beam Receive. First open up any new entry. In the Graffiti area, enter the shortcut key (lowercase cursive *L*), double tap, and enter *I*. This process will turn on Beam Receive for 5 seconds. This shortcut does not work with OS 4.

Applications. To access program options, tap Menu and then delete, beam, modify category, or find general information regarding each program. OS 4 will also copy programs from the main memory to SD cards or MMCs.

Synchronization. Be sure to specify how you want information to be updated on the PDA and desktop. The PDA can override the desktop, the desktop can override the PDA, or the two units can be synchronized to each other. The last option is the most widely used and is the default option. You can customize on a one-time or default basis the priority of the synchronization channels. Right click on the HotSync icon, and then go to the Custom selection. There you can modify the actions of each conduit as needed.

Essential Software

The following software will maximize productivity with your Palm OS PDA. In general, executable programs have the extension .prc, and most data have the extension .pdb or another extension (the extension depends on the program that created the data).

Document editors. In the Palm OS world, the standard document file is the doc file. This file type is similar to the Microsoft Word document type, and many programs support this file type. The advantage of document editors is that they eliminate the 4-KB file-size limit for memo files. In the practice of medicine, particularly psychiatry, the majority of information exchanged is text based. Hence, a document editor will be useful if you intend to do word processing.

Many companies have several versions of their programs. Some versions are free, allowing only viewing of doc files. The commercial versions offer editing and other functions. There are also IBM-compatible PC and Mac OS–based programs that permit text files and Microsoft Word files to be converted to Palm Doc format.

An increasing number of programs can directly convert Microsoft Word documents for editing on the Palm OS PDA. They all have basic font capabilities and paragraph styles but differ in the Menu display and in extra features. With each of these programs, you can beam documents to other users of the same program and print via the infrared transmitter when specific printing programs are used. Document editor options and differences are listed in Tables 5–2, 5–3, 5–4, and 5–5.

Spreadsheet programs.   Many programs synchronize with spreadsheet programs such as Microsoft Excel or connect to their own desktop spreadsheet counterparts. These programs (listed in Table 5–6) are capable of most of the complex functions of Microsoft Excel and offer formatting and other features. The disadvantage of spreadsheets on a PDA is that you must scroll to view all the cells.

Database programs.   These programs (see Table 5–7) are quite useful for creating your own patient database or synchronizing different forms with Microsoft Access or other open database connectivity (ODBC) databases. The choice of database software may be dependent on available third-party database files already created for specific patient-related tasks. For example, HanDBase offers a psychiatry record system. Check the Web site of the manufacturer, DDH Software (http://www.ddhsoftware.com), as well as http://www.memoware.com.

Database-form designers.   The programs listed in Table 5–8 facilitate creation of forms for inputting information. Many are quite sophisticated and allow separate application development.

Medical reference software.   Many medical texts are available for viewing on PDAs (see Table 5–9), including DSM-IV-TR (American Psychiatric Association 2000) and the American Psychiatric Association Practice Guidelines. Having such reference material on hand for review while on the move is a real convenience, but this ability does come with some caveats. Reading text on a PDA screen can be difficult. In addition, these texts take a large amount of memory, ranging from 742 KB *(The Massachusetts General Hospital Guide to Psychiatry in Primary Care)* to 4,048 KB or

TABLE 5–2. Document editing programs for Palm operating system personal digital assistants

Program	Web site	Doc	Microsoft Word	Memo	Miscellaneous	Printing program required
Documents To Go (Word To Go)	http://www.dataviz.com	No	Yes	No	Bundled with Palm, + PDF	IrPrint of InStep Print
WordSmith	http://www.bluenomad.com	Yes	Yes	Yes		PrintBoy or InStep Print
iambic Office (FastWriter)	http://www.iambic.com	Yes	Yes	Yes	+text files, RTF	Indirectly via PrintBoy "doc" printing
ThinkOffice (ThinkWord)	http://thinkingbytes.com	No	Yes	Yes		PrintBoy for ThinkOffice
QuickOffice (Quickword)	http://www.cesinc.com	Yes	Yes	Yes	Bundled with HandEra	PalmPrint or PrintBoy or InStep Print

Note. PDF=portable document format; RTF=rich text format.

TABLE 5–3. **Programs to enable printing from document editors**

Program	Web site	Feature
InStep Print	http://www.instepgroup.com	Can be used with InStep Fax
IrPrint	http://Doctoprint.irprint.com	DocToPrint specific for Documents To Go
PrintBoy	http://www.bachmannsoftware.com	Has suite compatible with many products
PalmPrint	http://www.stevenscreek.com	The first, but perhaps not as functional

4 MB *(The Merck Manual of Diagnosis and Therapy)*. Today, most Palm OS PDAs have 8 MB of main memory; Visor Pro has 16 MB. You can work around this limitation by adding memory. As described earlier, different external memory cards can be used, with capacities ranging from 8 to 256 MB, permitting storage of multiple digital texts.

The majority of the newer PDAs (e.g., Palm m500 and Palm m125, HandEra 330, Handspring PDAs, and Sony CLIÉ) have external expansion memory. The virtual file system used to access the external memory in Palm OS PDAs has a hitch. Although programs can be kept in the external memory card, when they are run they are actually copied to the main memory and run from there, only to be deleted from the main memory afterward. Most reference texts are data files to specific reader programs. Some reader programs can display the reference texts stored in the external memory while the reader program itself is in the main memory.

Programs to facilitate Mini-Mental State Exams. A few programs (listed in Table 5–10) facilitate the Mini-Mental State Exam by prompting the user with the questions and tasks. One program saves entries; another allows you to print the results.

Medication information software. These software packages (see Table 5–11) are quite popular and useful in busy practices.

TABLE 5–4. Document reading programs for Palm operating system personal digital assistants

Program	Web site	Additional file types	Miscellaneous
iSilo	http://www.isilo.com	HTML, iSilo format	Free version exists
iambic Reader	http://www.iambic.com/english/palmos/reader	Microsoft Word, HTML	
TealDoc	http://www.tealpoint.com/softdoc.htm	TealDoc	Popular
AportisDoc Mobile	http://www.aportis.com	Also supports PDF	Available for Pocket PC
ReadThemAll	http://www.Maksee.narod.ru/palm/rta/index.htm		Free, autoscrolling
Express Reader	http://www.qvadis.com/expressreader/pro.html		Free version: Lite
TomeRaider	http://www.tomeraider.com	TomeRaider specific	
CSpotRun	http://www.32768.com/bill/palmos/cspotrun/index.html		Free

Note. HTML = Hypertext Markup Language; PDF = Portable Document Format.

TABLE 5–5. **Document conversion programs for Palm operating system personal digital assistants**

Program	Web site	Feature
Screwdriver	http://pilot.screwdriver.net	URL (Web address) to Palm Doc format
MakeDocW	http://www.aportis.com/resources/AportisDoc/makedocutilities.html	Free, stand-alone program
pDocs	http://www.thinkchile.com/alorca	Incorporates as Microsoft Word menu

Some programs are electronic versions of paperback books, and others are products specifically created for the Palm OS platform. For example, Rx is a free pharmacology database from ePocrates that was created for the PDA. Rx has an update feature so that information remains current. In addition, it offers a multicheck feature, which allows the user to select several medications and then check for drug-drug interactions. It is one of two free drug guides available on the Internet; the other is the Tarascon ePharmacopoeia. Other programs such as *Physicians' Desk Reference* are available for purchase. The level of information varies, and it pays to download demonstration files to determine if the levels of information and detail are sufficient. Check http://www.handango.com, http://mobile.yahoo.com, and http://www.pdamd.com for prices.

Patient-tracking software. There are a variety of patient-tracking software packages available for general medicine (see Table 5–12) but few specifically geared toward psychiatry (see Table 5–13). Demonstration versions are available for most of the programs listed in Tables 5–12 and 5–13. Many of these programs, especially those in Table 5–12, have more features than you may need for organizing current patients in the hospital or in your practice.

Billing and coding software. Several billing and coding software packages are available (see Table 5–14). There are psychiatry versions of PocketBilling, a charge capture and tracking software program. Other packages are more general. Specific programs such

TABLE 5–6. Spreadsheet programs for Palm operating system personal digital assistants

Program	Web site	Microsoft Excel	Other types	Charting
Iambic Office (TinySheet)	http://www.iambic.com	Yes	No	Yes
Quickoffice (Quicksheet)	http://www.cesinc.com	Yes	No	Yes
ThinkOffice (ThinkSheet)	http://www.thinkingbytes.com	Yes	No	No
MiniCalc	http://www.solutionsinhand.com	Yes	No	Yes
Documents To Go (Sheet To Go)	http://www.dataviz.com	Yes	Lotus 1–2–3, Quattro Pro	No

TABLE 5–7. Database programs for Palm operating system personal digital assistants

Program	Web site	Microsoft Access	Additional features
thinkDB	http://www.thinkingbytes.com	Yes	Symbol scanner support, prints via PrintBoy
MobileDB	http://www.handmark.com	Yes	Microsoft Excel and FileMaker converters, which use PrintBoy PRO
HanDBase	http://www.ddhsoftware.com	Yes	Psychiatry record system available
JFile	http://www.land-j.com	Yes	Symbol scanner support, encryption

TABLE 5–8. Database form–designing programs for Palm operating system personal digital assistants

Program	Web site	Synchronization server	Other features
Pendragon Forms	http://www.pendragonsoftware.net	Yes	Internet forms
Kinectivity Studio	http://www.pencel.com	Yes	Tight control of data, synchronization, and exchange
Satellite Forms	http://www.pumatech.com	Yes	Many plug-ins for security, etc.
AppForge	http://www.appforge.com	No	Development platform
iAnywhere	http://www.ianywhere.com	Yes	Development solutions

TABLE 5–9. Medical reference software for Palm operating system personal digital assistants

Texts	Web site
DSM-IV-TR, American Psychiatric Association Practice Guidelines	http://www.appi.org
5-Minute Clinical Consult, DrDrugs, iFacts, Taber's Cyclopedic Medical Dictionary	http://www.skyscape.com
DSM-IV-TR, The Merck Manual of Diagnosis and Therapy, Harrison's Principles of Internal Medicine	http://www.handheldmed.com
The Merck Manual of Diagnosis and Therapy, Redi-Reference Clinical Guidelines	http://www.pdamd.com
See medical section	http://www.palmgear.com
Psych Dx, Psych Rx	http://www.medicalpiloteer.com
Clinical Psychiatry	http://www.handango.com
Files created by users and posted	http://www.memoware.com

TABLE 5–10. Mini-Mental State Exam programs for Palm operating system personal digital assistants

Program	Web site
Folstein Mini-Mental State Exam	http://www.nsbasic.com/pub/Palm_files/samples/Mmse.zip
miniMSE	http://www.medicalpiloteer.com
MentSTAT	http://www.tonywitte.com
MMSE Ir Print	http://www.tommybearsoftware.com/palmos.htm

as Stat E&M Coder assist with evaluation and management (E&M) coding, important for a consultation service.

Prescription-writing software.   Only a few companies currently offer prescription-writing software for Palm OS. When you use this software, you will be able to review different insurance plan formularies and will generate prescriptions in legible, machine-produced type. The Center for Primary Care Research at Johns Hopkins Uni-

TABLE 5–11. **Medication information software for Palm operating system personal digital assistants**

Programs	Web site
Rx	http://www.epocrates.com
A2zDrugs, DrDrugs	http://www.skyscape.com
Physicians' Desk Reference, The Medical Letter Handbook of Adverse Drug Interactions	http://www.franklin.com/pdr
Tarascon ePharmacopoeia	http://www.medscape.com

TABLE 5–12. **General patient–tracking programs for Palm operating system personal digital assistants**

Program	Web site
WardWatch	http://www.torlesse.com/pilot/wardwatch
Patient Tracker	http://www.handheldmed.com
Patient HandChart	http://www.ddhsoftware.com
PatientKeeper	http://www.patientkeeper.com

TABLE 5–13. **Psychiatric patient–tracking programs for Palm operating system personal digital assistants**

Program	Web site	Feature
Pocket Psychiatry	http://www.ddhsoftware.com	Uses HanDBase
Virtual Briefcase-Psych	http://www.thevirtualbriefcase.com	
SoapDish	http://www.ytechnology.com	

versity was recently funded by the Agency for Healthcare Research and Quality (2001) to study the effect of electronic prescriptions on medication errors.

ePhysician (http://www.ephysician.com) has an integrated software suite that both includes medication information and generates prescriptions. Prescriptions are sent to ePhysician via a wireless network or via an Internet connection when the PDA is synchro-

TABLE 5–14.   **Billing and coding programs for Palm operating system personal digital assistants**

Programs	Web site	Feature
ZapBill, ZapCode	http://www.zapmed.com	
Pocket Patient Billing	http://pocketpa.imrac.com	Psychiatry specialty version
PocketBilling	http://www.pocketmed.org	Psychiatry specialty version
Stat E&M Coder, Stat CPT	http://www.statcoder.com	Uses TealInfo

nized to a desktop computer. All prescriptions are sent directly from ePhysician to the appropriate pharmacy entered in the database.

Other companies offer the ability to print prescriptions directly from the PDA to a printer or to send them via fax when the PDA is synchronized. One company, iScribe (http://www.iscribe.com), offers its software free but requires that physicians upload their prescribing information to its Internet servers. iScribe's privacy statement is that any data are aggregated and that they do not provide individually identifiable data to any third party "other than in the context of medical treatment and payment." ScanRx, acquired by Salu (http://www.salu.com), also offers a printing-and-fax solution for purchase, without any sale of aggregated data.

Utilities and Functions

Beam and Move.   Palm OS does not allow you to beam certain copy-protected programs and information. This lock applies even to "free" programs, such as ePocrates qRx. Two programs—McFile and Filez—allow you to move your data or program files within your PDA, as well as exchange them with others. McFile is found at http://www.jade.dti.ne.jp/~imazeki/palm/McFl.index-e.html and Filez is available at http://www.nosleep.net.

Installation and Backup.   The standard method of installation in Palm OS PDAs is to use the Installation Tool, which utilizes the

HotSync conduit. When installing multiple files, you can avoid having to click on each file for installation or having to determine each file's location. When you specify that a program be installed, the program is copied into the Install folder located under your profile name (for example, C:\Palm\John\Install). Once the installation conduit has been activated in this manner, all you have to do is copy all the files you want to install into this folder. One drawback to installations is that all your conduits will be activated unless you modify the synchronization parameters.

In general, most users want to synchronize anyway, but doing so can be time consuming. A program called Pilot Install, available at http://www.pinstall.envicon.com, installs programs without invoking the synchronization conduits.

An advantage of synchronizing is that it creates backups of the programs and data. Although this is the default setting for the standard PDA features such as the address book, added software programs do not always back up either the programs or the data. For example, within QuickWord, you must specify which files should be backed up to the computer. With the program BackupBuddy, available from Blue Nomad (http://www.bluenomad.com), you can specify multiple backup actions, such as archiving deleted entries and backing up certain data and programs (including backup programs in flash memory and external memory).

HackMaster and Hacks.   Consider HackMaster (available at http://www.daggerware.com) a manager of patches that add extra features to the basic OS. HackMaster manages these system extensions in real time. Hacks are standardized extensions that add function, such as an extended find in all databases, or add additional "strokes" to carry out other activities. Most Hacks are available at http://www.palmgear.com and http://freewarepalm.com. X-Master (http://linkesoft.com) and EVPlugBase (http://freewarepalm.com) are free, compatible Hack managers that are newer and updated.

Hacks help you better use your Palm OS PDA. For example, FindHack will search all databases or selected databases, and Invert Hack will flip the pixels from dark-light and vice versa on monochrome PDAs. In general, these programs are not critical, but they add handy features to the PDA.

Security. The highly mobile nature of PDA use leaves PDAs vulnerable to theft and to risk of disclosure of private data. Patient information on a PDA must be secured. The best protection currently available is encryption software. Encryption of sensitive data on the Palm OS PDA works well and only minimally affects data access. There are other methods as well, including programs that limit access to certain applications containing sensitive data, and programs that force the user to enter a password for access. Other mechanisms such as user logs and hardware tokens are useful but can be rather burdensome. (See Chapter 9 for more discussion of security.) Some encryption options are listed in Table 5–15.

External Memory Access. Users of the older TRGpro Palm OS PDAs benefited from software that permitted them to access their external memory directly from the devices. Today, two programs are available to users of other Palm OS PDAs with external memory.

PowerRUN (http://www.tt.rim.or.jp/~tatsushi/index-e.html) frees up internal memory by allowing programs and data to be stored on the external memory card. PowerRUN moves the programs and data to the external memory card and keeps the necessary components stored in the internal memory. It works well for all programs except Hacks and anything requiring synchronization with the desktop computer.

TABLE 5–15. **Encryption programs for Palm operating system personal digital assistants**

Program	Web site
movianCrypt	http://www.moviansecurity.com
PDA Defense	http://www.pdadefense.com
PDASecure	http://www.trustdigital.com
FileCrypto	http://www.fsecure.com/wireless/palm/fc4palm

MSMount (http://www.geocities.com/nagamatu/MSMount/index-e.htm) works like PowerRUN, but users must manually move the programs using other programs such as McFile or Filez. MSMount establishes a mounting point for the programs in the internal memory. This tricks the PDA into thinking the programs are available in the internal memory, when the programs actually reside in the external memory.

Presentations.   Only two companies produce hardware or software for delivering presentations with the Palm OS PDA. MARGI Systems Presenter-to-Go (http://www.margi.com), a Handspring module and cable, allows the Handspring PDA to send slides to liquid crystal display (LCD) projectors or external monitors. It ships with software that will take any printed output and convert it for the presenter module. Web pages, documents, and Microsoft Power-Point slides can thus be "printed" to the PDA for display. Thus a computer is not needed for a presentation.

Synergy Solutions offers SlideShow Commander (http://www.synsolutions.com/software/slideshowcommander), which takes a different approach. Here, the slides remain on the computer. Instead of using the computer to control the presentation, this software uses the PDA. Speaker notes as well as the actual slide may be viewed on the PDA. The presenter may also highlight seconds of a slide on the PDA screen. This highlighted material will, in turn, be displayed by the LCD projector, eliminating the need for a laser pointer. Connection to the computer requires either a serial cable or a wireless Bluetooth or 802.11 interface.

Educational applications.   Training programs have adapted some of the aforementioned software and hardware for clinical and educational purposes.

The University of California at Davis Department of Psychiatry uses Palm OS PDAs to organize the consultation-liaison service (as described in Luo et al. 2001). With PDAs, portable keyboards, document editing software, and infrared printing software, the consultation team is able to generate progress notes. Documents are printed using a portable printer, eliminating the need to return to the department. In addition, electronic sign-out via PDA has been incorporated into the service. Using the to do list, the consultation team sends, via infrared beaming, a summary of patients to the "Consult PDA," which is then used by the weekend physician on rounds. On Monday, the weekday team transfers updated information regarding their individual patients back to their own PDAs of the regular consultation team.

At the Medical College of Wisconsin, PDAs are used to capture patient encounters as part of the resident logs. Formerly, Satellite Forms were used to generate data entry forms for the residents' PDAs. Now Pendragon Forms are used. The resident physicians then enter and submit these data to the main database by synchronizing their PDAs to a desktop computer. With Microsoft Access, both aggregate and individual reports are generated.

Pharmacology database programs have been extremely popular among residents at these two institutions.

Peripherals and Additional Software

There are numerous hardware devices for Palm OS PDAs. These hardware accessories enhance PDA functionality and connectivity. They may be specific to particular PDA models, because of the lack of standards for the serial port interface (where connections to cradles are made). Some accessories, as well as additional software, that are likely to be important for most users are covered here.

Keyboards. Several companies have created keyboards for Palm OS PDAs (see Table 5–16). One innovation is the folding keyboard, developed by Think Outside (http://www.thinkoutside.com). This keyboard starts to fold in a *W* pattern until it is only slightly larger than the PDA itself. Unfolded, the keyboard is nearly the size of a standard desktop keyboard. It is marketed by a variety of manufacturers, including Palm and Targus, for several PDAs. This keyboard is best for those who touch-type extensively.

Internet access mechanisms. There are several ways to access e-mail and the World Wide Web using a Palm OS PDA.

TABLE 5–16. Keyboards for Palm operating system personal digital assistants

Keyboard	Web sites	Features
Portable Keyboard	http://www.palm.com, http://www.targususa.com	Collapses to nearly PDA size, folds out to almost full size, must be used on flat surface (otherwise may malfunction)
GoType! Keyboard	http://www.landware.com	Small keys; rigid for use on lap
ThumbPad	http://www.targususa.com	Good for short entries, small, designed for thumb use only
Halfkeyboard	http://halfkeyboard.com	Very small; one-hand typing

Note. PDA=personal digital assistant.

Palm OS has its own mail program, but the program is not designed as an independent method to use e-mail. Rather, it is intended to be used with existing communication software through synchronization. After setup and pairing with an e-mail program such as Eudora or Outlook have occurred, e-mail will be downloaded, during synchronization, from your computer to your PDA for viewing whenever you wish. You may also prepare e-mail anytime; the program will save it until your next synchronization, when it will be loaded into your e-mail program for sending.

Another important product is AvantGo (http://www.avantgo.com), a Web site client. After establishing an account on this free service and installing the client software, you may select Web sites to be uploaded to your PDA from the AvantGo site. The content on these sites will be updated when you synchronize your PDA while your computer is connected live to the Internet. The pages have been specifically formatted for viewing on the PDA. You can specify others to be formatted by the AvantGo server. However, these may not translate well. ePocrates qRx uses this engine to update the drug information database. The software does not check the content on the device, only the synchronization date. Therefore, even if you have already updated content, the software will update again during synchronization, unless you have modified custom options.

To establish live connections to the Internet, most PDAs need modems. For example, there are modems for Palm Vx and Palm m500 to connect via regular telephone lines to Internet service providers, allowing for Web browsing and retrieval of e-mail. Some PDAs, such as Palm VIIx and the Handspring Treo, have built-in wireless modems; you pay a monthly service fee for Internet access. In addition, specific wireless data (modem) service, such as GoAmerica, OmniSky, and Sierra Wireless, can be obtained with the purchase of the appropriate modem. Check the available modems supported by the wireless provider. Some Palm OS PDAs can connect to the Internet via the infrared or wire-cable connection to a cellular telephone. However, data services are often a separate charge, so you must check with your cellular service provider. Connections offered by these services are still quite slow—up to 14.4 kilobits per second (Kbps), a rate that is best for text only. GPRS (General Packet Radio Service), which is on the horizon, will offer rates of up to 128 Kbps, but it will likely be available at first only to people in major metropolitan areas.

Web Sites

Numerous Web sites are dedicated to the Palm OS PDA. Those in Table 5–17 will provide you with links to all the products described earlier.

TABLE 5–17. **Useful Palm operating system personal digital assistant Web sites**

---

http://www.handango.com
http://www.palmgear.com
http://www.pdamd.com
http://www.eurocool.com
http://www.memoware.com
http://freewarepalm.com
http://www.hhcmag.com
http://www.pdabuzz.com
http://www.palmblvd.com

A popular e-mail discussion group for Palm OS PDA users in the medical field is Palm-Med (http://listserver.itd.umich.edu/cgi-bin/lyris.pl?enter=palm-med&text_mode=0&lang=english). To find other Web sites devoted to Palm OS PDAs and medical applications, go to http://www.medicalpiloteer.com and select Webring, or go to http://www.healthypalmpilot.com.

EPOC PDAs

Psion is the primary manufacturer of PDAs based on EPOC. However, in July 2001, the company announced that it had decided to focus on the industrial and enterprise markets. It will continue to make the existing PDAs for approximately a year (or longer, depending on demand), but it will not develop new models for consumers, because it found this area unprofitable. Current owners will be supported until December 2004, or longer if there is market demand. Two cellular telephone–PDA hybrids use EPOC: Nokia 9210 Communicator and Ericsson R380s.

Software

There are only a few developers of medical software for EPOC. Palmaris Medical (http://www.palmaris.com) markets several programs from these developers. ChartNote, for example, is a program to manage outpatients, and MediNotes is a database of medical information. Palmaris Medical also offers PdbRead, an EPOC Palm database reader. A few useful links are given in Table 5–18.

TABLE 5–18. **Useful EPOC personal digital assistant Web sites**

---

http://www.bjoern.com/s5_medic.htm
http://www.shanemckee.utvinternet.com
http://www.epocket.bizland.com/epocketdatabases
http://www.jwolfe.clara.net
http://www.symbcity.com
http://www.mydoktor.com
http://www.palmtop.co.uk
http://3lib.ukonline.co.uk

Pocket PC PDAs

In October 2001, Microsoft launched the latest version of its OS, Pocket PC 2002. This newer OS is significant not for its new features but for mandating standards regarding processor speed and screen size. Standardizing the central processing unit (CPU) means that developers no longer have to compile their software to run on specific devices; therefore, developing time and costs decrease. Having the speed of the processor standardized is also a benefit because software developers can rely on a standard capability of running programs. A standard screen size facilitates the appropriate display of information in this small form factor. For Pocket PC

2002, the standard CPU is an Intel 206-megahertz (MHz) StrongARM processor with a standard 32-MB ROM, and the display is a thin-film transistor (TFT) LCD of 240 × 320 pixels.

Deciding which Pocket PC device to use is complicated by the sheer number of devices available. Fortunately, with the new hardware standards, users may rely on more similarities than differences. As with the Palm OS PDAs, the main differences relate to expansion slots, form factor, and connectivity. On average, Pocket PC devices will run 8 hours per battery charge, depending on the application. If you can recharge often or carry an AC adapter, this is not an issue. However, if you are constantly on the go, a second, exchangeable battery may be necessary. Currently, Casio, Hewlett-Packard, and UR There International offer removable and interchangeable batteries. You can check http://www.pocketpc.com or the manufacturers' Web sites for details.

Bundled Software

All PDAs with Pocket PC 2002 ship with standard software (see Table 5–19). Many manufacturers include additional software on the compact disc (CD)–ROM or make more available at their Web sites.

Essential Software

Although the Pocket PC PDA is bundled with enough software for most users, you will need additional programs (listed in Table 5–20) to gain more function from your PDA. There are significantly fewer developers of software for Pocket PC than for Palm OS, but this is changing. Because Microsoft has standardized the CPU and screen size, developers can focus on one CPU instead of trying to support three different ones as with previous Pocket PC PDAs.

Medical Software

Every day there are more software titles for Pocket PC. Many of them are counterparts of software programs for Palm OS. Check Web sites such as http://www.handango.com, http://www.handheldmed.com,

TABLE 5–19. Software bundled with Pocket PC 2002 personal digital assistants

Software	Functions
Calendar	Appointment book, scheduler
Contacts	Telephone numbers, addresses, other contact information
Tasks	Organize and prioritize tasks
Inbox	Electronic mail
Pocket Internet Explorer	Web browser for Pocket PC
Pocket Word	Microsoft's word processing program, links to desktop documents
Pocket Excel	Microsoft's spreadsheet program, links to desktop documents
File Explorer	Copy, delete, and move files
Windows Media Player	Play video, MP3, and Microsoft audio format files
Terminal Server Client	Log into Windows NT Server with Terminal Server installed
Voice Recorder	Record and play short voice recordings
MSN Messenger	Microsoft's instant messenger program (live Internet connection required)
Microsoft Reader	eBook viewer with ClearType technology for easy reading
Notes	Jot down quick notes, link voice recordings
Microsoft Transcriber	Handwriting recognition program
Block Recognizer	Facilitate switching from Palm operating system to Pocket PC
ActiveSync	Synchronize Microsoft Outlook data with PDA, transfer and install files
Setup utilities	Configure communication settings, date, clock, etc.

Note. PDA=personal digital assistant.

TABLE 5–20. Essential Pocket PC programs

Program	Web site	Functions	Miscellaneous
PrintPocketCE	http://www.fieldsoftware.com	Enable printing of Pocket Word and transmission of e-mail via various mechanisms	Uses infrared, Bluetooth, LAN, serial, 802.11b connections to printers
Agenda Today	http://www.developerone.com	Enhanced schedule program	Many other useful utilities by developer
Task Pro Navigator	http://www.developerone.com	Application management tool	Very handy tool
Pocket Informant	http://www.pocketinformant.com	Integrated calendar, contact list, and task list	Many views of calendar
riteMail	http://ritemail.net	Exchange handwritten notes via e-mail	Useful for sending patients copies of any drawings made
Visual CE	http://www.syware.com	Create databases on PDA	mEnable gives wireless access to ODBC database
Handango Security Guard	http://www.handangosoftware.com	Encrypt folders and files	Needed for patient information
Pocket Connections Designer	http://www.pocketconnections.com	Rapid application-development tool	Also server and client software
Truefax	http://www.ksesoftware.com	Send and receive faxes	Creates fax from Pocket Outlook
HanDBase	http://www.ddhsoftware.com	Database program	

TABLE 5–20. Essential Pocket PC programs *(continued)*

Program	Web site	Functions	Miscellaneous
PocketSlides	http://www.conduits.com	View, edit, and display PowerPoint slides	External video card needed
Presenter-to-Go	http://www.margi.com	Display PowerPoint slides, but no transitions	Video with no extra card
CalliGrapher	http://www.phatware.com	Handwriting recognition	Upgraded Transcriber
Pocket Slide Show	http://www.cnetx.com	View, edit, and display PowerPoint slides	External video card needed
Peacemaker	http://www.conduits.com	Beam and receive from many infrared devices	Beam to Palm OS PDA, infrared equipped desktop or notebook

Note. e-mail=electronic mail; LAN=local area network; ODBC=open database connectivity; OS=operating system; PDA=personal digital assistant.

http://www.medicalpocketpc.com, and http://www.skyscape.com for these titles. Specific psychiatry reference texts such as *Psychiatric Drugs, The Massachusetts General Hospital Guide to Psychiatry in Primary Care, MGH Guide to Psychiatry in Primary Care,* and American Psychiatric Association Practice Guidelines are available. AportisDoc Mobile for Pocket PC can read Palm documents. An example of community discussion groups can be found at http://communities.msn.com/PocketPCMEd/_whatsnew.msnw.

There are numerous medical record systems, including Pock-etChart, Patient Tracker, and Mobile Med Data. Once again, these programs were written with other specialties in mind and offer more features than psychiatrists need. Eventually, there will be more medical software for Pocket PC, with links back to enterprise-wide data such as hospital electronic medical records. Until Palm produces PDAs with greater enterprise-computing capability (e.g., with faster CPUs, more addressable memory, and multimedia), Pocket PC is the platform to watch.

Peripherals

Many hardware accessories are available for Pocket PC PDAs, and most are interchangeable among different Pocket PC PDA makes because they fit SD/MMC, PCMCIA, or CF slots. Devices include bar code scanners, Ethernet cards, fax modems, random access memory (RAM), hard drives, and digital cameras. When deciding which device to buy, keep in mind that some devices may not fit into the expansion sleeves of your PDA. For example, Compact-Flash Type I is smaller than CompactFlash Type II. A useful resource for Pocket PC devices and software is *Pocket PC Magazine* (http://www.pocketpcmag.com).

■ REFERENCES

Agency for Healthcare Research and Quality: Using computers and information technology to prevent medical errors. Available at http://www.ahrq.gov/qual/newgrants/it.htm. Accessed December 16, 2001

American Psychiatric Association: Diagnostic and Statistical Manual of Mental Disorders, 4th Edition, Text Revision. Washington, DC, American Psychiatric Association, 2000

Luo J, Hales RE, Hilty DM, et al: Electronic sign-out using a personal digital assistant. Psychiatr Serv 52:173–174, 2001

SOFTWARE

Software is what makes hardware work. From the basic operating system (OS) to specific programs, software translates what you want to do into electrical signals that hardware understands. Having the right software makes it easier to accomplish your tasks.

■ OPERATING SYSTEM

In most computers, the OS is already installed. The OS is the software that controls and manages the daily functioning of your computer. It keeps track of all files, recognizes old and new computer components, handles all transfers of information from one part of your computer to another (e.g., transfers of information from your hard drive to your disk drive), and manages the assimilation and running of any software programs you purchase. Today, OSs also include utilities such as disk defragmenters, disk compression utilities, and Internet browsers.

Macintosh (Mac) computers use Apple OSs such as Mac OS X. That OS does not run on IBM-compatible personal computers (PCs), although there is software that can emulate an IBM-compatible unit OS in a Mac and hence run IBM-compatible PC software. Darwin, an open-source version of OS X for Intel x86 processors, may not support all IBM-compatible PC peripherals.

IBM-compatible computers, which make up the overwhelming majority of computers sold today, almost invariably run some version of Microsoft Windows. Some computers are sold with Linux, a free Unix-based alternative to Windows. Linux is favored by some serious computer users and programmers, but very little commercial software is currently available for consumers. Most Linux software is available at http://www.linux.org or other Web sites.

Microsoft generally makes OSs for the home or general consumer and corresponding OSs for business use. Although the two systems are similar, the business versions usually crash less frequently and have special networking and security features.

Windows 95, Windows 98, and Windows Me are the consumer versions and are still found on new computers being sold. Windows NT and Windows 2000 are still found on computers directed toward business. Windows XP is the newest Microsoft OS and reflects Microsoft's strategy to phase out the older MS-DOS based consumer lines and replace them with the more stable Windows NT kernel. In Windows XP the stability of Windows NT and Windows 2000 is merged with the user-friendly interface of Windows 95, Windows 98, and Windows Me.

Windows XP comes in a consumer version and a business version. The Windows startup interface has been modified, and a significant number of bells and whistles, including the OS's own brand of media player, have been added. Windows XP can be installed on only one computer; this feature was added to prevent piracy. After you have installed the OS, you must activate it via modem or the Internet. The OS is activated after Microsoft registers the configuration of your system (i.e., the components you have, such as a video card, the processor, and the hard drive) with your product identification number. If you do not activate Windows XP within 30 days of installation, you will be locked out of your system. If you change a significant number of components or install the OS on another machine, you will have to reactivate the OS.

In general, newer OSs are more expensive than older ones. Some older software and hardware may work with Windows 95 or Windows 98 but not with Windows 2000 or Windows NT. (For example, Windows NT does not support universal serial bus [USB] peripheral hardware.) Microsoft has announced that it will phase out support for Windows NT, so this particular OS should be avoided when making purchases. Many individuals and corporations refuse to purchase the latest OS. They prefer to wait for a revised edition or for a patch that fixes bugs or glitches that were not discovered before the launch of the new product. Typically, new computer OSs also require more memory, because they include more features.

■ TRADITIONAL SOFTWARE

Traditional software is defined here as software not specific to the practice of psychiatry but used by clinicians.

Word Processing Software

Very few secretaries still type dictation on typewriters. Word processing software, with its limitless capacity for revision and its spell checkers and grammar checkers, has made the typewriter and correction fluid virtually obsolete. Word processing software also allows you to change fonts and font sizes easily and, for example, reduce a 1½-page letter to 1 page. With this software, you can save time by copying text and graphics (e.g., charts, graphs, photos) from other sources, including the Internet, and then pasting them into the document you are working on. Storing documents in digital format also serves to supplement paper files.

Microsoft Word is the leading word processing program, followed by WordPerfect (Corel) and WordPro (Lotus). Numerous other programs are available commercially and as shareware or freeware. Shareware and freeware are software created by individuals and distributed free. In the case of shareware, if you find that the software is useful, you are expected to send a set payment to the creator. Shareware involves the honor system. Freeware, on the other hand, costs nothing whatsoever. Freeware and shareware can often be downloaded from the Internet. Most people choose word processing programs that they use at the office or that their friends have. Although many leading word processing programs translate documents from other formats, such translations are rarely perfect and often require some adjustment.

Spreadsheets

Spreadsheets are a valuable accounting tool. Budgeting office expenses and keeping track of clinical hours or travel or business expenses are tasks that can be facilitated with spreadsheets. A spreadsheet has a matrix of columns and rows where labels and numbers may be inserted. Mathematical formulas tabulate the raw data entered. Spreadsheets are perfect for answering "What if?" questions. For example, a spreadsheet with boxes summarizing business expenses and clinical revenues could answer the question "If I cut back my practice by 10%, how much would I have to cut back on expenses, or how much would I have to raise fees, to offset decreased earnings?"

Microsoft's spreadsheet is called Excel, and Corel produces Quattro Pro.

Database Software

Database programs permit filing and retrieval of information. Examples of these programs are on-line library catalogs and electronic address books. A clinician could keep a database of patients seen and include information on each patient, such as age, sex, diagnosis, medications prescribed, and global assessment of function scores at the beginning and end of treatment. Database software permits retrieval of each patient's information. It also permits you to answer questions such as "How many depressed male patients over 40 have I seen who have received a selective serotonin reuptake inhibitor?" or "What is the improvement in global assessment of function scores among my female patients with panic disorder?" A database of patient addresses might be used to generate mailing labels to announce the opening of a new office. Spreadsheets are also often used as databases and have numerous database features.

Microsoft produces Access and Visual FoxPro; Corel supports Paradox.

Presentation Software

Any psychiatrist or mental health professional who gives lectures or presentations to colleagues or the general public recognizes the importance of visual aids. Overhead transparencies, usually taking the form of slides, are a low-budget visual aid. Creating material for slides and bringing the material to a hospital's graphic design office or to an outside production firm usually results in costs of $9–$12 per slide. Presentation software allows you to construct your own slides. These slides may then be sent electronically or transported on a disk to a production firm. The cost per slide then decreases to $4–$5. If you have a notebook computer and a liquid crystal display (LCD) projector, no slides are needed, because you can project the images directly from the computer. Slides can be projected from a desktop computer as well, but carrying a desktop computer to the presentation site is awkward. The added advantage of presentation software is that slides may be changed right up to the moment of presentation. (For discussion of presentation programs and personal digital assistants, see Chapter 5.)

Internet Browsers

Connecting to the Internet requires an Internet service provider and software that enables you to capture the images that are floating on the information superhighway. The original mass-distributed browser, Netscape Navigator, can be obtained free at http://www.netscape.com. Microsoft bundled its browser, Internet Explorer, and has taken a commanding share of the browser market. Other browser software is available but is not as widely used as the two programs just mentioned. Opera (http://www.opera.com) is a shareware version noted for its speedy downloads and the small amount of memory it requires.

Electronic Mail Software

There are specialized programs for reading and storing electronic mail (e-mail). These programs allow you to create your own personalized address books and mailing lists. They also facilitate the reading and sending of attachments and can also filter out some unsolicited junk e-mail (spam).

Eudora, one of the original e-mail programs, can be obtained from the Internet either free (this version shows advertisements on the screen) or for a fee. (Check http://www.eudora.com.) Microsoft has bundled Outlook Express and Outlook with its software suites. (Software suites are discussed later in this chapter.)

Personal Information Managers

Date books, address books, and to do lists have been combined into software called personal information managers (PIMs). Frequently, these programs can be synchronized to personal digital assistants, permitting mobile viewing of information on the computer. E-mail may also be retrieved and accessed via the PIM. Palm Desktop and Microsoft Outlook are two PIMs (Outlook has bundled its e-mail program with its PIM).

Desktop Publishing Software

Desktop publishing programs provide an easy way to create announcements, posters, brochures, cards, banners, or anything else that is printed. You may mix and match fonts and insert clip art either from a library of images (both photos and illustrations) or from your own collection of images that you have scanned or photographed digitally. You can even print your own business cards, letterhead stationery, and envelopes. An office or practice newsletter is also easy to create and print. Microsoft Publisher is the best known of these programs. New word processing software also incorporates many desktop publishing features.

Web Page Design Software

Designing your own Web page used to involve learning a programming language called Hypertext Markup Language (HTML). Web page design software has simplified this process with drop and drag techniques similar to those used with all Windows-based software. After designing a Web page, you must contract with an Internet service provider to host your page (that is, place it on the Internet).

Programs in this category include Microsoft FrontPage, Adobe Web Collection, Macromedia Dreamweaver, and Fireworks Studio. If you have a Web page provided by a company such as Medem, you will not need a Web page design program, because you are not permitted to change the Web page yourself.

Software Suites

Almost all the programs discussed earlier in this chapter may be purchased individually. Software manufacturers have combined many of these programs into packages (suites). Buying the combination is significantly more economical than buying each component separately. Microsoft's newest suite is Office XP, Corel's latest suite is WordPerfect Office 2002, and Lotus now offers SmartSuite. The programs in Microsoft Works, a bare-bones suite, work fine, but they do not have all the features of more expensive collections.

Voice Recognition Software

Voice recognition software permits you to watch your words appear on the screen as you dictate. With this software, a large dictionary is stored in random access memory so that it is accessible when you speak into the microphone. As you speak, the speech engine attempts to match the words with those in the dictionary by making educated guesses based on sets of phonetic rules. A training period is required when the software is first installed, so that it can recognize and understand the specific pronunciation of the user, who might have a regional or foreign accent.

There are two kinds of voice recognition software: discrete and continuous. With the older style, discrete voice recognition software, you must pause after each word. It is very difficult to speak in this way. The newer version, continuous voice recognition software, allows you to speak normally. Significant breakthroughs in continuous voice recognition have resulted in a new set of capable and inexpensive computer programs.

The more you use such programs, the more accurate they become, because whenever an error occurs, the correction is stored for future reference. Accuracy reportedly approaches 90%. Some programs facilitate voice commands for basic computer functions. Most programs come with a 30,000- to 60,000-word vocabulary.

The two best-selling voice recognition programs are Dragon NaturallySpeaking and ViaVoice. Both programs sell for less than $150. Specialty medical modules have much larger professional vocabularies and may run an additional $500 or more.

Document Readers

Often information transmitted on the Internet is sent not as a word-processed file but as a graphic or picture. For example, if you wished to read a full-text journal article on-line, you might view either the words of the article or pages of the article as they appeared in the written journal. A document reader is required for you to do the latter. The most widely used document reader is Adobe Acrobat Reader, which can be downloaded free from http://www.adobe.com. To create documents for others to read, you must purchase Adobe Acrobat, available at the same site. eBooks also sometimes require a reader.

■ SPECIALIZED CLINICAL PROGRAMS

All the software discussed thus far is available either in stores or from mail-order companies, and the functions of these programs are adapted when used by mental health professionals. The following discussion relates to software designed with psychiatrists and other mental health professionals in mind.

Practice Management Software

Are you interested in a program that can take care of patient billing, track payments, submit claims electronically, schedule patient appointments, keep patient notes and treatment plans, and even assist in prescription writing and tracking? Practice management software performs various combinations of these tasks. Clinicians with programming skills have written some of this software. Some programs are geared toward solo or small practices, whereas others are designed to work on a local area network, for a large practice. A detailed review of earlier versions of this type of software is still in print (Rosen and Weil 1997).

Electronic Medical Record Software

Electronic medical record software is a step up from practice management software. Many of these systems are hospital based, and psychiatric modules are but one of many. These programs incorporate patient registration, admission examination, consultations, charting (by doctors, nurses, social workers, and others), laboratory results, medications, and everything else that used to reside in the patient's paper chart. This information can be entered at and retrieved from any computer terminal in the hospital. Some systems allow this information to be accessed from the doctor's outpatient office or clinic. Other systems allow the use of wireless handheld devices, which permit input and retrieval of data at the bedside.

There are usually multiple levels of security in such systems. One security measure is the registration of the date and time, the location of each computer terminal, and the name of each person who logs on to view the record. Progress notes may not be altered once they have been electronically signed. Among outpatient sites, patient information is usually transmitted along secured lines such as a virtual private network (VPN) or in encrypted files.

Most of these systems cost thousands, if not hundreds of thousands, of dollars. You can view a demonstration version of Sequest Technologies TIER (Totally Integrated Electronic Record) at http://www.sequest.net.

Psychological Testing Software

There are multiple programs that assist in administering, automating the scoring of, and interpreting results of psychological tests. It is not uncommon for clinics and private consultants to offer screening tools via computer to patients before the office visit or consultation. Some of these programs can simply organize a history, whereas others can be used to screen for depression, anxiety disorders, and other conditions.

Virtual Reality Software

Virtual reality permits an individual to step into a computer-generated three-dimensional world, either via a monitor screen or with special-effects goggles. Any movements by the viewer, who wears special gloves and other sensors, are incorporated into the virtual image. For example, a turn of the head will result in a corresponding change in the lines of sight. Although this technology has been used for games, it has also been incorporated into exposure and desensitization therapy for phobic disorders (Ackerman 1999).

Informational CD-ROMs

Psychiatry and psychology information is available on compact disc–read-only memory (CD-ROM). CD-ROM–based texts have not been particularly popular. American Psychiatric Publishing, Inc. (APPI) formerly published an electronic library on CD that included digital versions of its psychiatry textbooks and full-text journals. Now journal subscribers may access full-text versions of APPI's periodicals at http://www.psychiatryonline.org. Nonsubscribers can also search here for full-text articles and read them on a pay-per-view basis.

Other textbooks have included a CD-ROM version of the book. SilverPlatter (http://www.silverplatter.com) offers a CD-ROM database of psychiatric journal abstracts, updated quarterly, with Internet links to full texts. Pharmaceutical companies have provided a myriad of educational, multimedia CD-ROMs dealing with diagnosis, psychopharmacology, and neuroreceptors. With some programs, you can obtain continuing medical education credits.

Many of these CD-ROMs duplicate or supplement Internet resources. The advantages are their portability and the fact that you do not need an ongoing Internet connection to access the information.

Videoconferencing Software (and Hardware)

The ability to combine voice and video over plain old telephone system (POTS) lines has existed for years. New cameras and televisions and multiple Integrated Services Digital Network (ISDN) lines and software permit higher-resolution images that are of sufficient quality for a psychiatrist to observe movement disorders and for psychiatrists to conduct clinics miles from their patients. These systems (made by VTEL and PictureTel) cost $15,000–$30,000 per unit. Costs are decreasing. Low-priced alternatives (cameras costing less than $200) with software connections through the Internet can provide lower-resolution images sufficient for meetings and conversation but not for therapeutic work.

Bibliography Software

Bibliography software helps you organize references when you are writing an article or book. It also helps you download references from on-line databases and reformat the specific citations to conform to a particular publisher's criteria. The numerous software packages include Bookends Plus, EndNote Plus, and ProCite. A review of bibliography software can found at http://php.iupui.edu/ ~rsosborn/Scholars_Quest/References/Gathering/Reference_ Tools/Bibsoft-Guides&Resources.html.

■ UTILITY SOFTWARE

Utility software helps keep a computer running smoothly and efficiently. Many early utilities have now been incorporated into OSs, but many tasks remain that require, or are better performed by, additional software.

Antivirus Software

The increase in connectivity among computers has made them even more vulnerable to viruses. A computer virus can enter your computer through e-mail or Internet sites, as well as through files shared via floppy disks or other removable storage media. A virus may merely leave a message on your screen—or it may destroy data on your hard drive or send messages to everyone in your electronic address book, while spreading itself to the same group.

Antivirus software scans and detects known viruses and either eliminates them or alerts you to delete the contaminated files. Because new viruses appear daily, most programs provide the opportunity to update antivirus information each time you connect to the Internet. Examples of antivirus software include Norton AntiVirus, McAfee VirusScan, and PC-cillin.

Personal Firewall Software

Many institutions have constructed firewalls to prevent hackers from entering their computer systems via the Internet and engaging in mischief or sabotage. Many individuals now have Internet access through T1 or T3 lines or through DSL or cable modems and tend to leave their computers connected to the Internet for hours at a time. Individual computers thus become susceptible to hackers as well, who can take over a computer, delete files, or plant viruses directly. Personal firewall software provides a degree of protection against these intruders.

Free firewall programs for individual use include ZoneAlarm (http://www.zonealarm.com), Tiny Personal Firewall (http://www.tinysoftware.com/home/tiny), and Sygate Personal Firewall (http://www.free-firewall.org). A more robust version, ZoneAlarm Pro, is available for purchase at http://www.zonealarm.com. Symantec also sells Norton Personal Firewall (http://www.symantec.com/product). Other firewall software includes Network ICE Corporation's BlackICE Defender (http://www.networkice.com/products/soho_solutions.html) and McAfee Firewall (http://mcafeestore.beyond.com/FrontDoor/0,1076,3-18,00.html).

Other Utilities

System utilities perform automatic backups, check and seal off bad sectors of hard drives, help restore some deleted files, automatically defragment your hard drive, and do other functions. Some programs (e.g., Conversions Plus) help convert files from programs you do not own and allow you to open and read them. Other programs (e.g., MacDrive 2000) permit you to access files created on Macintosh computers and convert your files to Mac format.

■ REFERENCES

Ackerman JD: Virtual reality treatment for anxiety disorders. Paper presented at the annual meeting of the American College of Psychiatry, San Francisco, CA, February 1999

Rosen LD, Weil MM: The Mental Health Technology Bible. New York, Wiley, 1997

7

THE INTERNET

Nothing has changed the world of communications in the last decade as much as the Internet. Like the telephone, the Internet has had a tremendous impact on global communication. The Internet is still evolving as a communication and mass media network. Unlike television, it is an interactive medium: using the Internet, people can seek and interact with information. The Internet also includes new forms of information and new ways of looking at old information. It has truly made our world smaller and access to global resources easier.

The Internet was begun in the 1960s by the military, which wanted a computer communication network that could not be shut down. This network of networks was designed not with one main computer as director or coordinator but with each computer having the responsibility for communicating with the next one. In that way, if communication in one city was disrupted for any reason, there would not be disruption of the entire network. At the end of the Cold War, the military no longer needed these connections, and it turned the network over to universities and businesses. The infrastructure was in place; only further development was needed.

Most people believe that the World Wide Web is the Internet. It is not. The Internet is primarily composed of four elements: electronic mail (e-mail), the Web, file transfer protocol (FTP), and telnet (see Figure 7–1).

Telnet is the old mainframe-style, text-based protocol that made interactions difficult and frustrating. That is what the Internet looked like for several years. In 1990, Tim Berners-Lee decided that putting a graphic interface on the Internet would make it easy

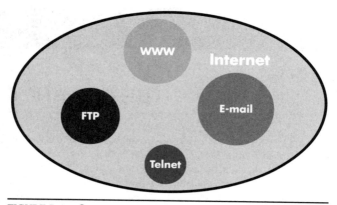

FIGURE 7–1. **Components of the Internet.**
Note. E-mail=electronic mail; FTP=File Transfer Protocol; www=World Wide Web.

for the user to point and click with a mouse to interact with the Internet. Thus the World Wide Web was born.

With software called a browser, the Web offers something that was previously unknown on the Internet: graphics, images, and sounds—that is, multimedia capabilities and the concepts of hyperlinks and hypertext. Hyperlinks allow a user to click on a word or graphic and "jump" to another Web page. In an instant, information is transported over the Internet to the user's computer.

FTP was devised to allow the transferring of files from one computer to another. FTP is generally the fastest way to send files over the Internet.

E-mail is a system for sending correspondence to anyone around the globe with an e-mail address.

■ E-MAIL

An e-mail message is an electronic document transmitted from a sender to one or more recipients. It is composed of a header and a body. The header contains a series of informative lines that tell the mailing system where to deliver the mail and that provide basic memorandum-like information for the sender and recipient or recipients. The body generally consists of text. However, it is possible to embed graphics, sound, and even full-motion video in the body of an e-mail message. See Figure 7–2 for an explanation of an e-mail address.

E-mail has become an important tool for collaboration. Keeping in touch with colleagues, sending reports for consultations, and organizing meetings can all be done using e-mail. It is virtually instantaneous. Documents, graphics, and pictures can be attached to the body of an e-mail message. Some clinicians use e-mail to correspond with patients.

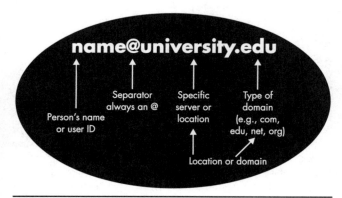

FIGURE 7–2. **Anatomy of an e-mail address.**

■ OTHER INTERACTIVE FEATURES ON THE INTERNET

E-Mail Discussion Groups

E-mail discussion groups are groups of people who collaborate or interact on a particular topic or theme using e-mail. These groups are generally private—that is, registration is required. A computer, or listserver, acts as a central processing center and gatekeeper for all e-mail communications among the group members, whose names and e-mail addresses make up a mailing list, and forwards all communications to all people on the list (Kramer and Kennedy 1998). One drawback of an e-mail discussion group is that members receive all communications within the group. Thus, a member may receive dozens of e-mail messages if there is lively discussion of a topic.

Newsgroups

Newsgroups permit public discussions on the Internet and are similar to public bulletin boards, in that messages are posted. After a message is posted to a newsgroup, anyone with software called a newsreader can post a response. Generally, newsgroups center around a topic and are open to anyone with Internet access.

Chat Rooms and Chat Groups

Chat is a popular form of immediate communication that takes place over the Internet and involves conferencing or bulletin board–type systems with real-time capabilities. Participants in chat rooms or chat groups engage in real-time conversation—that is, they type at the same time, as opposed to sending an e-mail message and then waiting for an e-mail response. Chat rooms or chat groups are offered by many on-line services. Hundreds or even thousands of users can be accommodated simultaneously. Some chat groups require special software, but most require only browsers. Chat rooms are generally topic driven.

■ CONNECTING TO THE INTERNET

There are in general two types of connections to the Internet: occasional connections (dial-up modem) and always-on connections (Integrated Services Digital Network [ISDN] cable, digital subscriber line [DSL], T1, and T3). Connection types and speeds are listed in

Table 7–1. The simplest way to connect to the Internet is through the plain old telephone system (POTS). Most home connections to the Internet are occasional, dial-up connections. The trend is toward always-on connections; millions of such connections are added to the roster of connections each year. The advantages of always-on connections are speed and instant access to the Internet.

TABLE 7–1.	**Connection types and speeds**	
Type of connection	**Download speed**	**Upload speed**
56K analog	56 Kbps or less	33.6 Kbps
ISDN	64 Kbps or 128 Kbps	64 Kbps or 128 Kbps
Cable	384 Kbps–4 Mbps	128 Kbps–4 Mbps
DSL	144 Kbps–8 Mbps	144 Kbps–1.7 Mbps
T1	1.54 Mbps	1.54 Mbps
T3	44.736 Mbps	44.736 Mbps

Note. DSL=digital subscriber line; ISDN=Integrated Services Digital Network; Kbps=kilobits per second; Mbps=megabits per second.

To connect to the Internet, an Internet service provider (ISP) is needed. The ISP is connected to the Internet with an always-on connection, and dialing in through a telephone line gives the average home computer user e-mail and access to the Web and the rest of the Internet.

The majority of business and university connections to the Internet are always-on, high-speed connections (e.g., T1) and are made available to all the various users through a local area network. This makes it possible for a large number of people to have speedy connections to the Internet. It also allows for an intranet, a closed private system for sharing information.

See Figure 7–3 for an explanation of an Internet, or Web, address.

■ BROWSING

Browsing is a search strategy that can be very effective. To browse, you start at a Web site that is likely to lead you to your specific area

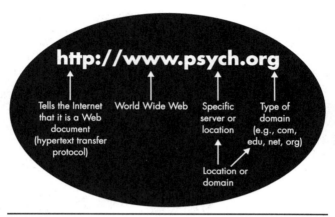

FIGURE 7–3. **Anatomy of a Web address.**

of interest. For example, you might begin at the American Psychiatric Association Web site: www.psych.org. As you scroll through
the site, you will notice that when your mouse pointer turns into a
hand or when text is underlined or in color, you are able to click on
the graphic or text where the pointer is located. These areas are
known as hot links or hypertext links. From your starting site, you
click on interesting-looking hot links or hypertext links, which lead
you to another document within that site or to a different site alto-
gether. You continue in this fashion until you find the information
you need.

■ ACCESSING INFORMATION
ON THE INTERNET

The Internet is not organized into a single index. According to Pool
(1994), "the Internet is like a library without a card catalog." It is
composed of billions of Web pages and other types of information,
and there is no central way to locate any particular page or piece of

information. Search engines help people navigate this ocean of information. These programs cull information from the Internet and organize it into logical, hierarchical, searchable lists.

There are essentially three categories of search indices or programs: spiders or Web crawlers, catalogs, and hybrids. Spiders are small programs that traverse the Internet looking for Web sites. When they locate a site, they index virtually every word they find and every link they come across. This results in an index of words, phrases, and connections. Catalogs are created by people. If you create a Web site, you submit the URL (Web address) and a description of your site to the catalog, and the catalogers decide whether to include it. Generally, catalogs include only the index page or home page of a site. More specific searches are possible through a catalog because it is usually organized and filtered for duplicates, but a catalog does not know if sites are changed or updated. Hybrids combine spiders and catalogs and thus result in more accurate searches. Metasearch engines do not have their own databases but search other databases and return your query from other sites.

Search Techniques

It is important to learn the particulars of how a search engine works. It is helpful to read the search tips on the respective sites, because you will find out how a particular engine handles searches that include more than one word. Most search engines return results that include any of the words. Because there is so much information online, you will probably want to limit your searches. Limiting and refining your searches can be accomplished using Boolean operators. Boolean logic uses operators to determine whether a statement is true or false. The most common operators are *AND, OR,* and *NOT.* These three words can be quite important when doing on-line searches (see Table 7–2).

In some searches, the case of the letters (i.e., uppercase or lowercase) of the search terms matters. It may also be possible to search by phrases or by date. At many search sites, the most common or popular searches are organized into easy-to-assess lists.

TABLE 7–2.	Results of searches with common Boolean operators
Search phrase	**Search result**
computerized testing	Pages containing both words are listed first, followed by pages containing only one of the two words.
computerized AND testing, + computerized + testing	Both words must appear somewhere on the page.
computerized + testing	*Computerized* must be on the page; *testing* should be.
+ testing – computerized, testing NOT computerized	*Computerized testing* must be on the page; *computerized* must not.
"computerized testing"	*Computerized testing* must appear as a phrase on the page.
computerized*	Phrases that start with *computerized* (e.g., *computerized assessment, computerized homes*) appear on the page.

Selecting Information

The Internet is a democracy. That is, anyone can create a site and place any information that he or she wishes on it. Bad poetry, doctoral dissertations, and anything in between—all have equal importance. A search can produce a vast array of results; thus, the more specific the search, the better the search result. For example, a search using the word *depression* may bring up information on the DSM-IV-TR (American Psychiatric Association 2000) diagnostic criteria for depression but will also provide you with information on the Great Depression of the 1930s.

Integrity of Information

Information obtained on-line can be of many types and can come from many places around the globe. An issue confronting the average consumer is how to determine the integrity and quality of information presented on the Web. Because all things are equal on the Web, the user should beware. The amount of information is staggering, and the results obtained by browsing can be overwhelming. Information such as medical information is offered easily and freely (for the cost of banner ads), and it is difficult for the average reader to determine whether the data presented are factual and whether the writer or site has the credentials to present high-quality medical information.

■ PSYCHIATRY AND THE INTERNET

Psychiatry and mental health hold special interest on the Internet for many people—consumers as well as professionals. Twenty-six percent of people looking for health information on-line are seeking mental health information ("The Online Health Care Revolution" 2001). Extensive information on psychiatry is available, ranging from simple guides to complex algorithms to on-line support groups to sites offering advice. Clearly, sites offering mental health information need to be viewed with a critical eye. Psychiatrists (and other mental health professionals) need to be aware of the sites that are publicly available because their patients are inevitably going to mention sites to them, ask for suggestions, or come to their psychiatrists' offices with printouts from psychiatry-related Web sites.

Virtually every university and hospital in the United States has Web sites that describe their programs and services. Many also provide information for consumers. When universities and publishers realized the power and global reach of the Web, they began making their research and publications available on the Web. On-line versions of the important journals initially supplemented the printed versions. Currently, the move is toward offering more on-line than paper versions. The Web allows for new ways of publishing and new approaches to providing academicians, clinicians, and researchers with valuable published information.

Many associations, societies, and professional organizations also have Web sites. The journals of some of these organizations are available on-line. In the last decade, there has been debate about whether these on-line journals should be free. The current trend is to offer the abstracts at no charge but to require a paid subscription and registration on the Web site for access to entire articles. However, many books and journals are available free on-line.

The same is true with regard to continuing medical education (CME) on-line. Some sites charge a nominal fee and others offer CME for free. In addition to Web sites of professional associations, a number of on-line "megasites" offer daily news, original peer-reviewed articles, articles from paper journals, conference reports, and CME. Examples of these sites are included in Table 7–3.

■ REFERENCES

American Psychiatric Association: Diagnostic and Statistical Manual of Mental Disorders, 4th Edition, Text Revision. Washington, DC, American Psychiatric Association, 2000

The online health care revolution: how the Web helps Americans take better care of themselves. The Pew Internet & American Life Project. Available at: http://www.pewinternet.org/reports/toc.asp?Report=26. Accessed December 3, 2001

Kramer T, Kennedy R: The World Wide Web and Internet: on-line communication, collaboration, and collegiality. Acad Psychiatry 22:66–69, 1998

Pool R: Turning adn info-glut into a library. Science 266:20–22, 1994

TABLE 7–3. Clinically relevant Internet Web sites

Resource	Web site
Associations and societies	
Academy of Psychosomatic Medicine	http://www.apm.org
Administrators in Academic Psychiatry	http://www.adminpsych.org/aap.htm
American Academy of Addiction Psychiatry	http://www.aaap.org
American Academy of Child and Adolescent Psychiatry	http://www.aacap.org
American Academy of Psychiatry and the Law	http://www.aapl.org
American Association of Directors of Psychiatric Residency Training	http://www.aadprt.org
American Association for Geriatric Psychiatry	http://www.aagpgpa.org
American Neuropsychiatric Association	http://www.neuropsychiatry.com/ANPA/index.html
American Psychiatric Association	http://www.psych.org
American Psychiatric Publishing, Inc.	http://www.appi.org
American Psychosomatic Society	http://www.psychosomatic.org
American Psychoanalytic Association	http://apsa.org
American Psychological Association	http://www.apa.org
Association for Academic Psychiatry	http://www.hsc.wvu.edu/aap/home.htm
Canadian Psychiatric Association	http://www.cpa-apc.org
Freud Net: The A A Brill Library	http://www.nypsa.org
National Alliance for the Mentally Ill	http://www.nami.org
National Institute of Mental Health	http://www.nimh.nih.gov
National Mental Health Association	http://www.nmha.org
Society of Biological Psychiatry	http://www.sobp.org

TABLE 7–3. Clinically relevant Internet Web sites *(continued)*

Resource	Web site
Substance Abuse and Mental Health Services Administration	http://www.samhsa.gov
World Health Organization: International Statistical Classification of Diseases	http://www.who.int/whosis/icd10
General psychiatry and continuing medical education (CME)	
American Medical Association Freida Online (residency programs)	http://www.ama-assn.org/ama/pub/category/2997.html
CME-CE.com	http://www.cme-ce.com
CME conference index	http://www.mhsource.com/conf/index.html
CMEweb	http://www.cmeweb.com
Dr. Bob's Mental Health Links	http://www.dr-bob.org/mental.html
HospitalWeb (Web sites of various hospitals)	http://neuro-www.mgh.harvard.edu/hospitalweb.shtml
Medscape Psychiatry & Mental Health (information and CME)	http://psychiatry.medscape.com
MedWeb—Emory University	http://www.medweb.emory.edu/MedWeb
Mental Health InfoSource	http://www.mhsource.com
Mental health meeting, organization, and resource index	http://www.umdnj.edu/psyevnts/psyjumps.html
National Institute of Mental Health	http://www.nimh.nih.gov
National Institutes of Health News & Events	http://www.nih.gov/news/
National Institutes of Health CME	http://odp.od.nih.gov/consensus/cme/cme.htm
Online CME listing (B Sklar, MD)	http://netcantina.com/bernardsklar
Psychiatry Residency Programs	http://www.webcom.com/wooming/residenc/psych.html
Virtual Medical Law Center	http://www-sci.lib.uci.edu/HSG/L.egal.html

TABLE 7–3.   Clinically relevant Internet Web sites *(continued)*

Resource	Web site
General mental health resources and consumer information	
American Psychiatric Association Public Information	http://www.psych.org/public_info
Behavior OnLine	http://www.behavior.net
Help! A Consumer's Guide to Mental Health Information	http://www.vex.net/~madmagic/help/help.html
Internet Mental Health	http://www.mentalhealth.com
Mental health associations listing (Mental Health InfoSource)	http://www.mhsource.com/hy/address.html
Mental Health Foundation (United Kingdom)	http://www.mentalhealth.org.uk
Mental Health InfoSource	http://www.mhsource.com
NetPsychology	http://netpsych.com
Psych Central Dr. Grohol's Mental Health Page	http://www.psychcentral.com
Royal College of Psychiatrists "Help is at Hand" leaflet series	http://www.rcpsych.ac.uk/info/help/index.htm
Pharmaceutical and drug information	
Clinical Pharmacology Online	http://www.cponline.gsm.com
Food and Drug Administration	http://www.fda.gov
Health*touch*—Drug Information	http://www.healthtouch.com/level1/p_dri.htm
Psychopharmacology Tips by Dr. Bob	http://www.dr-bob.org/tips
RxList	http://www.rxlist.com
USP (U.S. Pharmacopeia)	http://www.usp.org
Journals	
Extensive list of journals in psychology and mental health and social science	http://www.psycline.org/journals/psycline.html
Journals of American Psychiatric Publishing, Inc.	http://psychiatryonline.org

TABLE 7–3. Clinically relevant Internet Web sites *(continued)*

Resource	Web site
American Journal of Psychiatry	http://ajp.psychiatryonline.org
Archives of General Psychiatry	http://archpsyc.ama-assn.org
Canadian Journal of Psychiatry	http://www.cpa-apc.org/Publications/Publications.asp
Journal of Clinical Psychiatry	http://www.psychiatrist.com
New England Journal of Medicine	http://www.nejm.org
Psychiatric Times	http://www.psychiatrictimes.com
Psychwatch listing of psychiatry journals around the world	http://www.psychwatch.com/psychiatry_journals.htm
Research	
CenterWatch Clinical Trials Listing Service	http://www.centerwatch.com
Interactive Testing in Psychiatry—New York University Dept. of Psychiatry (board-style questions and annotated answers on-line)	http://www.med.nyu.edu/Psych/itp.html
NIMH Research Web sites	http://www.nimh.nih.gov/research/nimhwebs.cfm
Neuropsychiatry	
Neurosciences on the Internet (searchable database and extensive resources)	http://www.neuroguide.com/
Schedules for Clinical Assessment in Neuropsychiatry	http://www.who.int/m/topics/scan/en
Computers and informatics	
American Medical Informatics Association	http://www.amia.org
Catalyst (information on computers in psychology)	http://www.victoriapoint.com/catalyst.htm
Computers in Mental Health	http://www.ex.ac.uk/cimh
Psychiatric Society for Informatics	http://www.psych.med.umich.edu/
Yale Telemedicine Center	http://info.med.yale.edu/telmed

TABLE 7–3. Clinically relevant Internet Web sites *(continued)*

Resource	Web site
MEDLINE	
MEDLINE	http://www.ncbi.nlm.nih.gov/PubMed
MEDLINEplus (topic driven)	http://www.nlm.nih.gov/medlineplus
PubMed Central (archive of life sciences journal literature)	http://www.pubmedcentral.nih.gov
Medical sites	
American Medical Association	http://www.ama-assn.org
DIRLINE: Directory of Health Organizations	http://dirline.nlm.nih.gov
Doctor's Guide	http://www.docguide.com
eMedicine (eMedicine journal and World Medical Library)	http://www.emedicine.com
Medical Matrix	http://www.medmatrix.org
Medscape	http://www.medscape.com
Merck Manual of Diagnosis and Therapy	http://www.merck.com/pubs/mmanual
National Institutes of Health	http://www.nih.gov
National Library of Medicine	http://www.nlm.nih.gov
On-line Medical Dictionary	http://www.graylab.ac.uk/omd/index.html
Virtual Hospital	http://www.vh.org
Virtual Hospital online textbooks	http://www.vh.org/Providers/Textbooks/MultimediaTextbooks.html

TABLE 7–3. Clinically relevant Internet Web sites *(continued)*

Resource	Web site
Consumer medical sites	
MedicineNet Diseases & Conditions/Procedures & Tests; Medications; and Dictionary	http://www.medicinenet.com
National electronic Library for Health (United Kingdom)	http://www.nelh.nhs.uk
WebMD Health	http://my.webmd.com
Popular search engines	
AltaVista Search	http://altavista.com
Dogpile (metasearch engine)	http://www.dogpile.com
Excite: Mental Health	http://excite.healthology.com
Four11 (Yahoo people search)	http://www.four11.com
Google	http://www.google.com
HealthAtoZ	http://www.HealthAtoZ.com
HotBot	http://www.hotbot.com
Medsite (medical information, books, and software)	http://www.medsite.com
Multisearch engine	http://www.metacrawler.com
On-line language translation	http://world.altavista.com
Search.com (metasearch engine)	http://www.search.com
Search Engine Watch (tips and information on searches)	http://searchenginewatch.com
Switchboard (telephone and address directory)	http://www.switchboard.com
WhoWhere (index of personal Web pages, Internet yellow pages, and e-mail addresses)	http://www.whowhere.com

TABLE 7–3.   Clinically relevant Internet Web sites *(continued)*

Resource	Web site
Yahoo: Mental Health	http://dir.yahoo.com/Health/Mental_Health
Other search engines	
About	http://www.about.com
Excite	http://www.excite.com
LookSmart	http://www.looksmart.com
Lycos	http://www.lycos.com
Web sites on specific conditions	
Alcohol dependence	
Al-Anon and Alateen	http://www.al-anon.alateen.org
Alcoholics Anonymous	http://www.alcoholics-anonymous.org
Online AA Recovery Resources	http://www.recovery.org/aa
Alzheimer's disease	
Alzheimer's Association	http://www.alz.org
Anxiety disorders	
Anxiety Disorders Association of America	http://www.adaa.org
Anxiety Panic Internet Resource	http://www.algy.com/anxiety
CyberPsych Anxiety Disorders Links	http://www.cyberpsych.org/anxlink.htm#pd
Panic/Anxiety Disorders Guide at the Mining Company	http://panicdisorder.miningco.com
Attention-deficit disorders	
Children and Adults With Attention-Deficit/Disorder	http://www.chadd.org
National Attention Deficit Disorder Association	http://www.add.org

TABLE 7–3.   Clinically relevant Internet Web sites *(continued)*

Resource	Web site
Autism	
Autism Society of America	http://www.autism-society.org
Conditions in children and adolescents	
The Arc	http://www.thearc.org
Learning Disabilities Association of America	http://www.ldanatl.org
Online Asperger Syndrome Information & Support	http://www.udel.edu/bkirby/asperger
Pediatric Psychiatry Pamphlets	http://www.klis.com/chandler
Dissociation	
International Society for the Study of Dissociation	http://www.issd.org
Sidran Traumatic Stress Institute	http://www.sidran.org
Eating disorders	
ANRED: Anorexia Nervosa and Related Eating Disorders	http://www.anred.com
National Eating Disorders Association	http://www.NationalEatingDisorders.org)
Something Fishy Website on Eating Disorders	http://www.something-fishy.org
Factitious disorders	
Dr. Marc Feldman's Munchausen Syndrome, Factitious Disorder, and Munchausen by Proxy Page	http://www.munchausen.com

TABLE 7–3. Clinically relevant Internet Web sites *(continued)*

Resource	Web site
Mood disorders	
Depression.com	http://www.depression.com
Depression Guide at the Mining Company	http://depression.miningco.com
Dr. Ivan's Depression Central	http://www.psycom.net/depression.central.html
National Depressive and Manic/Depressive Association	http://www.ndmda.org
Nicotine dependence	
Arizona Smokers' Helpline	http://www.ashline.org
QuitNet (resource to quit smoking)	http://www.quitnet.org
Obsessive-compulsive disorders	
Obsessive-Compulsive Foundation	http://www.ocfoundation.org
OC & Spectrum Disorders Association	http://www.ocdhelp.org
Personality disorders	
Avoidant Personality Group Homepage	http://www.geocities.com/HotSprings/3764
BPD Central (borderline personality disorder)	http://www.BPDCentral.com
Schizophrenia	
Schizophrenia.com	http://www.schizophrenia.com
Schizophrenia Digest	http://www.vaxxine.com/schizophrenia
Sexual disorders	
Society for Human Sexuality	http://www.sexuality.org

TABLE 7–3. Clinically relevant Internet Web sites *(continued)*

Resource	Web site
Sleep disorders	
Sleep Medicine Home Page	http://www.cloud9.net/~thorpy
Sleepnet.com Tips for Healthy Sleep	http://www.sleepnet.com
Somatoform disorders	
Somatoform disorders	http://campus.houghton.edu/depts/psychology/abn7a
Substance-related disorders	
Addiction Resource Guide	http://www.hubplace.com/addiction
Cocaine Anonymous	http://www.ca.org
National Institute on Drug Abuse	http://www.nida.nih.gov
PREVLINE: National Clearinghouse for Alcohol and Drug Information	http://www.health.org
Substance Abuse and Mental Health Services Administration	http://www.samhsa.gov
Web of Addictions	http://www.well.com/user/woa
Tourette syndrome	
Tourette Syndrome Association	http://www.tsa-usa.org
Traumatic stress–related conditions	
International Society for Traumatic Stress Studies	http://www.istss.org
National Center for PTSD (includes PILOTS database)	http://www.ncptsd.org

8

TELEMEDICINE

The term *telemedicine* commonly refers to videoconferencing. However, telemedicine encompasses all technologies related to the practice of medicine at a distance, including electronic mail (e-mail), voice mail, faxes, and even the telephone.

There are increasing uses for these technologies in the practice of medicine today. Telemedicine is used more and more often because of the limited access that many people have to mental health services. Initially, the barriers to telemedicine were primarily technology and cost, because the hardware requirements were significant. Today, with faster Internet connections available to the general public and decreasing costs of video equipment, telemedicine is poised to be an important tool in clinical practice.

■ APPLICATIONS

Telemedicine has been used to provide direct health services to people in rural, suburban, and urban areas. It is also quite useful for providing specialist consultations from academic medical centers to facilities in areas with physician shortages. In such cases, the primary physician collaborates with the consulting psychiatrist. Services also can be delivered to specific populations. For example, a psychiatrist fluent in American Sign Language may "visit" his or her hearing-impaired clients via telemedicine (Craft 1996). In the past, that psychiatrist would have spent half the day traveling to see a few patients, but now visits can be more regularly scheduled.

At the Veterans Affairs hospital in Milwaukee, Wisconsin, staff psychiatrists conduct a weekly psychopharmacology clinic for patients at the Veterans Affairs hospital in Iron Mountain, Michigan, more than 200 miles away. In Kearney, Nebraska, psychiatrists evaluate patients, prescribe medications, and conduct predischarge planning on site and use telemedicine to provide postdischarge follow-up and psychotherapy. Initially, two "hubs" in the general and psychiatric hospitals in Kearney connected to "spoke" hospitals in five distant communities. A third hub was added in the emergency department of the general hospital, and five additional community hospitals have joined the system (J. Berlin, personal communication, October 2001).

This technology is not limited to patient care. It permits remote supervision as well as attendance at educational conferences. At the University of California at Davis, regular physicians' group meetings are held in both Sacramento and Davis, because a large number of physicians practice in both areas. Teleconferencing connects physicians at the two sites.

E-mail is used as a means of communication between provider and patient. It is fast and relatively easy to use, and in some instances it has replaced regular mail. At the annual meeting of the Psychiatric Society for Informatics, Yager (2000) presented his use of e-mail to extend communication with his eating disorder patients in rural New Mexico. The patients found it difficult to travel for several hours on a regular basis for appointments. E-mail facilitated follow-up. Both he and his patients were satisfied with the mode of communication.

■ NECESSARY TECHNOLOGY

Telemedicine relies on fast and reliable connections. For good video quality, 30 frames per second is the minimum refresh rate, and a frequency of 4 kilohertz (KHz) is desirable for telephone-quality audio. Initially, Integrated Services Digital Network (ISDN) was the only way to ensure adequate bandwidth for transmission of video and audio signals. Regular analog modems are limited to 56 kilobits per second (Kbps), an insufficient bandwidth, and they are unreliable. Although operating systems such as Windows 98 allow for multiple modems to be used in parallel over plain old telephone system (POTS) lines, this is not a reliable solution relative to other technologies.

ISDN provides for a direct connection similar to that achieved with telephone lines. It consists of two channels, A and B, at 128 Kbps each and an additional sideband, which is used to relay channel information. The advantage of ISDN is that both channels can be combined to provide a rate of 384 Kbps, the speed that allows adequate audio and video transmission without too much lag or signal breakup. Although ISDN is a fairly reliable and steady service, it has several disadvantages. Availability is a key issue; many small towns and remote areas do not have a telecommunications provider willing to supply services. In addition, costs are high, because special lines are needed to transmit at these speeds. Despite these limitations, ISDN has been the established standard in telemedicine, and some states, such as Wisconsin, have mandated that utilities provide ISDN lines to the doors of hospitals and schools throughout the state.

Many areas now have more broadband options. DSL is an increasingly popular and relatively inexpensive method for fast Internet access using regular phone lines. Most telecommunication companies advertise a downstream-transmission rate of up to 1.5 megabits per second (Mbps), but the speed is dependent both on the distance between your home or office and the switching station and on the condition of telephone lines. In addition, it is important to purchase a plan with adequate upstream- and downstream-transmission speeds. Many of the currently advertised prices are for business or home users who typically download (receive) information more than they upload (send) information.

Cable modems are another broadband option for obtaining fast Internet access. In general, cable modems permit faster transmission than does DSL. However, a cable modem connection is not an individual connection; all cable modems share the same bandwidth.

Hence, if there are too many users, the actual transmission speed may be significantly decreased.

Another alternative for remote areas is a two-way very small aperture terminal (VSAT) satellite connection. This service, which was launched in 2000, provides for speeds up to 10 times faster than those of a dial-up modem. Although the bandwidth is adequate with this service, there is a 0.5- to 1-second delay in video, which disrupts the flow. Satellite transmissions may also be interrupted by inclement weather.

The technology includes the ability to remotely tilt and pan the camera, as well as zoom and focus. The microphone system must be sufficiently sensitive to transmit the nuances of speech. Video camera suites have been expensive. Not long ago, you could spend $50,000–$75,000 per unit. Although prices have decreased considerably, these suites are likely still rather expensive for the individual physician. Small, desktop cameras are not adequate for clinical videoconferencing, because their resolution and refresh rate are too poor for good results. In the future, you will be able to connect your television and DSL or cable modem line to provide telemedicine services.

In general, most sessions are interactive, requiring the simultaneous presence of both parties. These sessions require the most bandwidth, in order to have adequate-quality video and audio. However, when interaction is not necessary, such as in educational vignettes, store-and-forward technology is used. The speed of connection in these circumstances is not critical, because the video and audio are stored in a file, which is sent to the user.

As mentioned earlier, ISDN is the established standard in telemedicine. One reason for this is that it uses a direct connection between the two computers, thereby preventing unauthorized access to the session. When you use DSL or a cable modem, the video and audio are sent as "packets," which are small chunks of the data. It is possible, though not easy, to capture these packets and thus gain access to the video and audio. Therefore, if data are to be sent over the Internet, a virtual private network (VPN) should be established.

■ OBSTACLES TO IMPLEMENTATION

Technology is not the only hurdle to overcome in telemedicine. A major concern relates to medical licensing. Today, if a physician in Nevada wishes to see a patient in California, he or she must have a license in California. The physician must be licensed in the state where the patient is located, because practice of medicine is considered to occur in the state where the patient resides. It has been proposed that a national license for the practice of telemedicine be created. State medical licensing boards, however, do not wish to relinquish their authority and cannot agree on details such as which state would have jurisdiction for review.

Another significant problem in telemedicine is the handling of emergency situations. The distant treating physician may not know what emergency resources are available to the patient, and telemedicine will be considered the culprit if an unfavorable event occurs. It is good practice to have established policies regarding emergency contact and to have a local physician available for a suicidal patient. The American Psychiatric Association (1998) produced a resource document on telemedicine policies.

The reliability of telemedicine for patient care is yet another concern. Depending on video quality, the physician may misinterpret certain symptoms or conditions such as extrapyramidal symptoms or tardive dyskinesia. Research assessing the ability of the Brief Psychiatric Rating Scale in telemedicine versus direct care has demonstrated good interrater reliability (Baigent et al. 1997). However, when patients with schizophrenia were evaluated, via telemedicine, using the Positive and Negative Syndrome Scale for Schizophrenia, positive symptoms were well identified but negative symptoms were more difficult to assess (Zarate et al. 1997).

The telemedicine medium also affects the patient-physician relationship. Patients have found the audio portion to be more important than the video portion in terms of conveying the sense of information exchange (Cukor et al. 1998). Zarate et al. (1997) discovered that the majority of schizophrenia patients studied actually preferred telemedicine to direct care.

Much of the research regarding telemedicine has demonstrated fairly good patient and provider satisfaction (Mair and Whitten 2000). Many variables affect satisfaction, including comfort with technology, age, travel distance, and waiting time. Many psychiatrists express concern about the effect of technology on establishing a relationship and rapport (Dongier et al. 1986).

E-mail used in clinical situations is associated with similar issues regarding privacy, policies, and satisfaction. Special guidelines concerning privacy have been established and include recognizing identifiable information as highly sensitive; providing safeguards based on fair information practices; empowering patients by providing information and granting the right to consent to disclosure; limiting disclosures of health data absent consent; and incorporating industry-wide security protections (Hodge et al. 1999). The American Medical Informatics Association has developed guidelines for the use of e-mail, including obtaining informed consent before using e-mail, explaining the security mechanisms used, prohibiting the forwarding of patient e-mail without express authorization, informing patients about anyone who has access to records, responsibly responding to messages, and avoiding references to third parties (Kane and Sands 1998).

■ REFERENCES

American Psychiatric Association: APA resource document on telepsychiatry via videoconferencing. Available at: http://www.psych.org/pract_of_psych/tp_paper.cfm. Accessed December 23, 2001

Baigent MF, Lloyd CJ, Kavanagh SJ, et al: Telepsychiatry: "tele" yes, but what about the "psychiatry"? J Telemed Telecare 3:3–5, 1997

Craft SH: Telemedicine Services: Serving Deaf Clients Through Cutting-Edge Technology. Columbia, SC, South Carolina Department of Mental Health, 1996

Cukor P, Baer L, Willis BS, et al: Use of videophones and low-cost standard telephone lines to provide a social presence in telepsychiatry. Telemed J 4:313–321, 1998

Dongier M, Tempier R, Lalinec-Michaud M, et al: Telepsychiatry: psychiatric consultation through two-way television. a controlled study. Can J Psychiatry 31:32–34, 1986

Hodge JG, Gostin LO, Jacobson PD: Legal issues concerning electronic health information: privacy, quality, and liability. JAMA 282:1466–1471, 1999

Kane B, Sands DZ: Guidelines for the clinical use of electronic mail with patients. The AMIA Internet Working Group, Task Force on Guidelines for the Use of Clinic-Patient Electronic Mail. J Am Med Inform Assoc 5:104–111, 1998

Mair F, Whitten P: Systematic review of studies of patient satisfaction with telemedicine. BMJ 320:1517–1520, 2000

Yager J: E-mail as a therapeutic adjunct in the outpatient treatment of anorexia nervosa: illustrative case material and discussion of the issues. Paper presented at the annual meeting of the Psychiatric Society for Informatics, Chicago, IL, May 2000

Zarate CA, Weinstock L, Cukor P, et al: Applicability of telemedicine for assessing patients with schizophrenia: acceptance and reliability. J Clin Psychiatry 58:22–25, 1997

9

SECURITY

Computer use in the practice of psychiatry is associated with a number of security issues, including patient confidentiality, integrity, and information availability. Policies and technology must prevent unauthorized access to data in any electronic device or system.

■ HEALTH INFORMATION PORTABILITY AND ACCOUNTABILITY ACT OF 1996

The purpose of the Health Information Portability and Accountability Act of 1996 (HIPAA) is to improve the efficiency and effectiveness of electronic information. It mandates that all providers who bill electronically (directly or through clearinghouses) implement security measures in these transactions, to maintain the privacy of an individual's medical record. There are other provisions as well, including measures regarding how and when providers may release information. Providers must disclose to whom information is released, and violators are held accountable. Information in electronic form is easily transmitted, intentionally and unintentionally; thus, security measures must be instituted. HIPAA is scheduled to take effect in 2003.

The data covered by this act are any protected health information, such as records related to a person's health, provision of care, or payment. Also included are patient identifiers, information created by or received from a HIPAA-covered entity, and any information electronically generated, maintained, or transmitted. The information itself is protected, not just the record in which it appears.

The focus of HIPAA is on individuals' rights. Patients have the right to written notice of information practices from health plans and providers; the right to inspect and copy their protected health information; the right to request amendment or correction; the right to an accounting of disclosures for purposes other than treatment, payment, or health care operations; and the right to complain to a covered entity or the Department of Health and Human Services.

A key concept is the minimum necessary rule, which states that providers must disclose only that information necessary to accomplish the purpose of disclosure. HIPAA does not mandate any particular security mechanism, but there are clear penalties for any breach of its provisions. Penalties take the form of fines (ranging from $50,000 to $250,000 for each occurrence) and prison terms (of up to 10 years). The "minimum necessary" scope indicates that the security mechanism implemented be reasonably appropriate to limit inadvertent or unnecessary disclosure of information. The security mechanism need not be excessive. For example, it may not be necessary for X-ray light boxes to be isolated, but they should not be accessible to the public.

■ SECURITY POLICIES

Appropriate security policies must be in place, and certain protocols must be enacted when there is a security breach. It may not be necessary for a private practice to have a security officer, but within a group practice, someone should be designated as the person in charge. Policies should include the statement that any unnecessary access to patient information will result in dismissal. Staff and physicians should sign a security agreement, indicating that they understand the policy.

■ SECURITY MEASURES TO CONTROL AND MONITOR ACCESS

Access can be controlled and monitored in a variety of ways (see Table 9–1). On a desktop or laptop computer, sensitive files should be encrypted. This mechanism is the most secure, although it can be defeated with too simple a password (a password is needed for decoding). Ideally, a tracking program should be installed, to keep track of who uses the computer and also which files were accessed and when they were accessed. Changes to the medical record must be recorded, so that attempts to modify data are also known. When the user leaves the computer, he or she should log off so that no one else can take advantage of his or her access level. In the future, a token such as a key card may be required, in conjunction with the password, to gain access.

TABLE 9–1.   **Security measures**

Location	Security measure	Function
Computer	Encryption	Prevent unauthorized viewing of data
Computer	Password	Prevent unauthorized computer access
Computer	Access logs	Track who is accessing certain files
Computer	Password-enabled screen saver	Prevent unauthorized access
Electronic mail	Encryption	Prevent unauthorized viewing of messages
Internet	Firewalls	Prevent unauthorized access to computer files

Passwords are a simple, effective mechanism to control access. However, when a password is written down and stuck on a computer, it is useless. Ideally, passwords should have at least six characters, with some symbols and/or numbers, and should not include meaningful words such as the name of a pet or spouse. Sharing passwords is common but should be discouraged. Passwords should be changed on a regular basis.

All modern computers have built-in system passwords. These passwords are disabled by default. If you wish to use your computer password, find how to access the system password or BIOS password in your computer manual. When the computer is first booted up, you will see several messages on the screen. Typically, one message will be an instruction to hit a certain key to access the BIOS. Once you are in the BIOS setup, you can specify the system password. Write the password down and keep it in a secure location; you will not be able to start the computer without it.

Biometric hardware, another means of access control, is becoming more reliable and affordable. Instead of a password, a fingerprint or retinal scan is used to gain access. Many of these scanners are integrated into mice and keyboards. If a user is not permitted access after fingerprint or retinal scanning, a password is requested.

You may control access to computers by setting up user accounts. One person must manage the accounts and set up privileges for other users. Users of operating systems such as Windows 2000 and Windows XP are required to have accounts to gain access. Windows 95 and Window 98 do not have this security feature, and the login is easily bypassed. Computers connected to a network using Novell NetWare or Windows NT also require user accounts, which log access to the local area network. It is a good habit to log out of your account when finished. Doing so will prevent others from accessing data using your account.

If you must leave the computer on for a short period, block access to the computer with a password-enabled screen saver. Although this mechanism is not an absolute security measure, it is a deterrent to anyone trying to snoop or send messages in your name. Kane and Sands (1998) recommend that you not only make your electronic mail (e-mail) program password enabled but log out of the program when not using it.

■ INTERNET SECURITY MEASURES

When connected to the Internet, you must pay attention to what you are doing. For example, it is easy to send an e-mail message to the wrong person or to disclose information to an e-mail discussion group. E-mail has all the privacy of a postcard. Patients should be told not to disclose any sensitive information when communicating with their physicians via e-mail (Kane and Sands 1998). Patients should also know when e-mail will be answered and should be instructed to use the subject line. Providers should not use personal e-mail accounts for business; it is better to keep accounts separate, to avoid accidental disclosure. The e-mail client program should be password protected, and providers should exit the program when done, so that others cannot view sensitive information or send messages inappropriately.

Computers connected to the Internet should have firewall software (see section "Personal Firewall Software" in Chapter 6 of this book). These programs prevent designated outside programs from sending information to and gaining information from a computer network.

■ HARDWARE SECURITY MEASURES

Protect your investment and, more importantly, protect your data. Unfortunately, there is quite a market for stolen computers of any type, and chances are that about a day after your personal computer (PC) is stolen, it will be halfway across the country. Notebooks are the most likely to be stolen, primarily because of their size, but desktop PCs and various peripherals are also vulnerable. Anything that can be grabbed and stuffed in a duffel bag should be cabled or otherwise secured to a desk.

Mark your equipment. Engrave your name, driver's license number, and other identifying data, and keep a list of your serial numbers. You might wish to identify yourself or your company in your AUTOEXEC.BAT. (This file is used by Windows OS computers to start the computer.) Why? If your computer ends up several hundred miles away, purchased by someone who thinks that it is a new or reconditioned PC, the buyer will be alerted that it belongs to you, and you might possibly get the computer back.

A wire cable is a popular means of securing a desktop computer in an office. The cable is braided wire with a loop at each end. A ring is glued to the PC, and another ring is glued to the desk; then the cable is run through the rings, and the ends of the cable are locked with a padlock. Although someone with a very good set of wire cutters could cut the cable, many thefts are impulsive grabs of pieces of equipment, and the cable would deter such a theft.

Another method of securing your desktop PC is to use security plates. A bottom plate is bolted to the desktop, and a second plate is either bolted or glued to the PC. These plates prevent theft quite well, but if you decide to change desks or redecorate your office, you will find them almost impossible to remove. If you are successful in removing them, large chunks of desktop or computer will come as well.

Peripherals may be stolen, too. Add-on peripherals are easy targets. Zip drives, small scanners, tape drives—anything that is small enough to fit into a travel bag is at risk. Store these items in a secure location.

If you own a notebook computer, be conscious of where it is. Do not leave it in an empty office or conference room, even for a couple of minutes. It takes less than 5 seconds for someone to grab it and hide it in a briefcase or bag. If you must leave your notebook for a short period, use a motion sensor. This device has a retractable cable that facilitates attachment to the notebook. Any movement sets off a shrieking alarm. Do not leave your notebook in the backseat of your car, and do not leave it in your hotel room. Use the hotel safety deposit box or, if one is provided, an in-room safe. Travelers carrying notebook computers are favorite targets for theft. Just as you would protect a pocketbook or important bag, take appropriate precautions when carrying a notebook in an airport or busy commuter terminal. Security checkpoints are notorious locations for losing notebook computers. While the owner is passing through the metal detector and is physically separated from the notebook, someone else is walking off with the scanned computer. Concealing your notebook in something that is not obviously a computer case is a partial deterrent.

■ REFERENCES

Health Care Financing Administration: HIPAA insurance reform. Available at: www.hcfa.gov/medicaid/hipaa/default.asp. Accessed December 21, 2001

Kane B, Sands DZ: Guidelines for the clinical use of electronic mail with patients. The AMIA Internet Working Group, Task Force on Guidelines for the Use of Clinic-Patient Electronic Mail. J Am Med Inform Assoc 5:104–111, 1998

10

MAINTENANCE, PREVENTION, AND TIPS

This chapter contains miscellaneous information that novice computers users may find helpful. Although these recommendations appear to be common sense, they are not often followed.

■ STARTING UP

Every time you turn on your computer, it performs a series of tests on each of the system's major circuits. It then tests its memory, disk drives, keyboard, screen, and internal chips. If everything is working properly, your familiar desktop screen appears.

This warm-up procedure is called a power-on self test (POST). The only signs that a POST is in progress are the sounds of floppy disks turning briefly, a single beep to confirm that at least some of the computer is working well, and a pause while the computer checks its memory.

If there are problems at this early phase, you may hear multiple beeps, signifying that something is wrong. This could be something as simple as the need for a new internal battery or the fact that you did not plug in your keyboard, or it could be something more serious, such as problems with memory or other hardware problems. You should write down the error message that appears.

The first thing to do when troubleshooting your computer is to make sure that it is plugged in and getting proper power. It is not unusual for a computer technician to make an expensive house call for a computer that the owner thinks is broken but that in actuality is not plugged in. In other instances, the monitor is reported as being blown out when it has been turned off or when the contrast or brightness has been reduced. Also, if a device was recently connected, check that the pins on the connector are not bent. This holds true for anything you plug into the computer. Make sure all cables (e.g., printer, modem, and monitor cables) are plugged into the computer and into a power source. When in doubt, read the instruction manual!

■ MINIMIZING WEAR AND TEAR

Using your computer imposes normal wear and tear on its components. Following these few general rules will help make your computer last longer.

Do not turn your computer on and off frequently.   If you use the computer at different times throughout the day, leave it on between these periods of use. It is better for the computer to stay on than to be turned on and off repeatedly.

Clean your floppy disk drives regularly.   Generally, clean your floppy disk drive with a head cleaner monthly. If the computer is in a dusty or smoky environment, clean it more frequently.

Run hard drive (hard disk) utilities regularly.   To maintain hard disk speed and integrity, you should run disk utilities such as Scan-Disk, which comes with Windows. These utilities clean up lost files and reorganize the files on your hard drive so that it runs faster. They also detect and repair early hard disk damage. Remember, hard drives do not last forever, and they *all* start to show some wear and damage. Back up your important files regularly!

■ BACKING UP

Backing up is the process of copying your files to something other than your hard drive. If you turn on your computer one day and it no longer works, you still have a copy of your files, if you have backed them up. You can then move to another computer and resume working. If your hard disk crashes, you can always reinstall your favorite word processing program using the original disks, but you may not be able to get to your own files if you do not have a backup.

Because you can never completely avoid problems with your computer, you should have copies of any programs or data files that are important. The saying "An ounce of prevention is worth a pound of cure" certainly applies to computers. Backing up regularly is the only way to prevent loss.

Many people ask, "How often should I back up my data?" The answer is "How much are you willing to lose?" In response to this, most people say, "Nothing." To avoid losing anything whatsoever, you would have to back up every minute. Obviously, this is not practical. Most offices generally back up at the end of the day. If you are writing an important report or paper, you may wish to back up every 15–30 minutes. Keep a copy on an alternative media source such as a floppy disk or a compact disc–rewritable (CD-RW).

The simplest way to back up is to copy your files to a floppy disk. Large data files such as digital photos require larger storage media. Commercial backup programs, which are widely available and relatively inexpensive, automate the backup process and offer more backup methods. For example, a program may allow you to back up only those files created since the last time you backed up, or all files ending in .doc, or you could back up to a tape drive automatically at a certain time of day. Some backup programs compress data so that the data take up less space.

At home, the easiest way to back up your personal computer (PC) is to copy your data files to a floppy disk (labeled "Backup") at least daily. Doing so will ensure that there is a second copy of your documents. Many word processing programs make short-term backups, called timed backups, which are backups to your hard drive that are made automatically every 10 minutes (or at any interval you specify). This feature is useful if you have a power failure or someone accidentally unplugs your computer and files are deleted when you exit the program. You can recapture your files from the last timed backup.

Businesses that need to back up large amounts of data files invest in tape drives for backup, or they copy to removable hard disks and store the backups in a safe place. Many businesses adopt an alternating-backup method, backing up on tape number 1 on Monday, tape number 2 on Tuesday, and so on. If there is a computer problem and files are damaged, data can be retrieved from a previous day's backup tape. This method is also particularly helpful if a computer virus is discovered that may have been on the computer for a couple of days before causing problems. CD-RW burners are now commonplace on desktop and notebook computers. They are also a useful backup medium, but if you require more than 650-megabyte (MB) capacity, a tape backup system may be needed.

■ PREVENTING DISASTERS

The following are tips to prevent computer disasters.

Create an emergency disk.   No PC user should be without an emergency disk that contains the files needed to start the system again. Many PCs come with an emergency CD or disk containing the system files needed to restore your computer to a functional state in the event of problems. You can also create an emergency startup disk by following the instructions in the Add/Remove Programs section of your operating system. Once you create the disk, label it plainly, date it, and keep it close to your PC at all times, either near your desktop computer or with your portable when you are on the road.

Back up faithfully.   It cannot be said enough: Backing up the data on your computer is one of the easiest and most effective forms of preventive maintenance. Yet even computer users with the best of intentions often skip backups in their haste to move on to the next project. It is not until they lose hours, or even days, of work that they wish they had spent the few minutes it takes to create a backup.

Here is one backup strategy: Once a week, back up your entire hard disk. Every day, make an incremental backup of new files and those that have changed since they were last backed up. You should also perform a full backup before making any system changes.

Keep your backups in a safe place, and when it is time to make the next one, do not overwrite the previous version. Use a different tape or disk so that you have another on hand in case something goes wrong. And if your system has multiple drives, make sure you are backing up all of them.

Defragment.   If your hard disk seems to be getting slower and slower, it is time to defragment. Files are stored in bits and pieces in different locations on your hard disk. Hard disk heads must search the entire surface of the drive to reconstruct an entire file. Defragmentation takes all the separate fragments of a file and physically repositions them onto one contiguous segment. This reduces head movement and improves performance.

Many programs have a quick-optimization feature that cleans up the major fragmentation in a matter of minutes. However, full-fledged disk optimization can take as long as several hours, depending on the size of your hard disk. If you are a heavy user and frequently work with lots of small files, you should probably do a complete defragmentation of your hard disk about once a month.

The newest generation of optimizers can work automatically in Windows. Many of these programs offer various options. For example, you can have the program watch your hard disk for fragmentation and have it automatically optimize when fragmentation reaches a certain level. You can even set it to optimize overnight, so that your system is not bogged down while you are in the middle of a hectic workday.

Play it safe. Defragmenters rarely cause problems, but you should make a full backup of your hard disk before defragmenting, just in case.

Eliminate clutter.   Uninstalling software is not always as simple as installing it. Many installation programs scatter bits and pieces of applications in ini files (initiation files that set up Windows starting parameters) and in other places you would never think of looking. That can slow down your system, because Windows reads every line in its ini files every time the computer starts up.

Using a product such as UnInstaller, an uninstall utility, can help you find the files you do not need, along with all their widely scattered bits and pieces. UnInstaller will also check for duplicate files and orphans (files that are not necessary for installed applications). However, do not indiscriminately delete files just because a utility has put them on the orphan list. First make sure that the files are not critical to any of your applications.

Consider using technical support.   Many hardware or software manufacturers provide technical support for a limited time after you purchase a product. Depending on the product, this can be a godsend or a nightmare. Some manufacturers provide toll-free numbers; others make you pay for the call. In either case, you should be prepared to be on hold for some length of time.

The number for technical support can usually be found in the first few pages of the manual that comes with your purchase. Before calling, you should have in front of you the information that the technical support person needs, such as the serial number, make, or model of the computer; the version of the software; or the configuration of your system. The more the staff person knows, the faster he or she can solve your problem. Many people are intimidated by technology, and everyone is afraid of asking stupid questions, but most technical support staff have heard it all before.

■ UPDATING

Many new versions of computer programs offer new or improved features or fixes of bugs found after the programs were marketed. Updating programs can therefore be useful. Improvements and fixes are also included in new versions of files called drivers, which help the operating system communicate with or operate peripherals, such as a mouse or a floppy disk drive. In general, if your computer is running well, it may not be necessary to buy the latest drivers, but they may improve speed or stability. It is hard to keep up with all the versions of software.

A very good Internet-based update service is CatchUp (http://catchup.cnet.com), which is free. You start by downloading a program that allows the Internet server to survey your hard drive for all your drivers and software programs. There are two checks: one for the most recent versions of software and drivers, and the other for security vulnerabilities. After a scan, the Web site displays a list of the programs or drivers that may need to be updated, and you can then download and install them at your discretion.

■ INSURING YOUR COMPUTER

There are companies that will insure your computer equipment. You may also wish to check with your automobile, homeowners, or renters insurance company; you may be able to cover your computer equipment as well, for a small additional fee.

Safeware was one of the first companies to insure computer equipment. Insurance is quite inexpensive, and the coverage is quite extensive. One precaution: save all your receipts. Your only viable proof of ownership is your purchase receipt. If your equipment is stolen, call the police and make a record of it. You need to have a record of the theft and the events surrounding it to process your insurance claim.

■ SUMMARY

By following the advice in this chapter, you can reduce your anxiety about potential problems. Even experts cannot avoid having hard drive failures or monitor burnouts. Backing up and updating your computer will ensure that you will survive any unforeseen emergencies.

11

THE FUTURE

"The future isn't what it used to be," wrote the French poet Paul Valéry (1964). This is probably more true than one ever would have believed. The influence of technology has been extremely strong in the last decade. Things formerly considered futuristic have been developed or occurred so quickly that even defining the present has been a difficult task.

In the last decade, it has become clear that technology can enhance the understanding and practice of psychiatry. Technology will certainly become easier, faster, smaller, and smarter. As the hardware becomes more capable, smarter programs will be developed in areas such as speech recognition, in which the ability to understand the spoken word and to speak back to the user will improve dramatically. In addition, speech recognition software will be used not only in desktop and notebook computers but in personal digital assistants (PDAs) as well.

How has this development of technology affected psychiatry?

■ THE INTERNET

Studies show that 90% of physicians are connected to the Internet (Pastore 2001). Over the last decade, individuals, professional associations, academic institutions, and clinical facilities have been populating the World Wide Web and adding a wealth of information. Web sites dedicated to psychiatry and mental health have blossomed during this period of "Web building," and there is certainly a plethora of on-line journals, articles, books, and clinical algorithms.

Because the Internet has become such a pervasive and important medium, all other technologies will use the Internet for connection, communication, and interaction. As the Internet becomes ubiquitous, so will technology. What people call the Internet today will become just "the network." All types of connections will be used.

■ OTHER TECHNOLOGIES

Other computer technologies have begun to affect the practice of psychiatry. Consider the following scenario:

> Dr. Alfred Jones starts his day. The Internet appliance sitting on his breakfast table is part of the wireless network that connects numerous computers and other appliances in his home. He orally asks his home computer to show him his schedule for the day and then has it read aloud the neurological report that he has just received from a consultant on one of his patients. Finally, he reviews the morning newspaper on-screen.
>
> During his morning commute to the office, he instructs his PDA to reschedule a meeting and synchronize the schedules of the six members of an education committee. He then review bills electronically and authorizes payment and then instructs the PDA to make dinner reservations for that evening to celebrate his anniversary.
>
> Dr. Jones later arrives at his university medical center to make ward rounds with his residents. In the nursing station, his PDA downloads the current charts of all the patients whose cases he will review with his trainees. As he walks around the ward, he can review the charts, order tests, change medications, and complete treatment plans. These changes are uploaded to the hospital computer at the end of his rounds.

Clinicians want technology to do what they already do—only better and faster. The technology to accomplish these complex tasks already exists. Implementation will take place over the next decade.

■ ELECTRONIC MEDICAL RECORDS

Web-enabled electronic medical records (EMRs), also known as digital health records (DHR) or computerized patient record (CPR), have been a health care goal for more than a decade. From the beginning, the Internet has been governed by a set of communication standards and protocols. These established guidelines make it a logical platform upon which to build a health care information system that can be universally adopted.

Using a Web-accessible format, clinicians can instantaneously access all the usual elements of a medical record. In addition, there are options and information that only an electronic medium can offer, such as error checking, formulary information, insurance and coding information, and constantly updated links to sites with the latest clinical and pharmacological information. All this information is also available in abbreviated format via mobile phone or PDA with wireless capability. The Health Information Portability and Accountability Act of 1996 (HIPAA) will hasten the arrival of EMRs, not because HIPAA mandates the use of EMRs, but because with EMRs, it will be easier to comply with requirements such as tracking everyone who has accessed a patient chart.

Patients' involvement with their medical records will increase in the years to come as EMRs become standard. Patients will interact easily and freely with their own EMRs and their physicians, leading to patient empowerment and improved patient-physician communication. Patients want to manage more of their health care from home, and they can do so. At the physician's Web site, appointments can be made and insurance information can be reviewed. Patients can review their EMRs to obtain laboratory test results or other information.

■ PATIENT SCREENING

Some psychopharmacology consultants ask patients to complete computer screening forms before coming to the office for consultations. At several outpatient clinics, patients complete scan forms during registration. These forms include a depression screen and other clinical scales. A number of consultation-liaison services use scan forms or PDAs to input clinical information obtained during consultations. These are samples of future trends. Such clinical tools can be used to supplement findings of diagnostic interviews or consultations.

■ TREATMENT

Can computer technology become a part of psychiatric treatment? It certainly will not replace treatment, but it can supplement treatment in specific ways. A computer program called OCD-Trainer, developed in Germany, gives patients daily activities to complete, to assist them in gaining control over compulsive rituals (Wölk 2001). The computer can handle repetitive tasks very well, never tiring or becoming bored, and the patient can have access at any time of day.

Telepsychiatry is an important and viable supplement to clinical assessment and treatment, especially in rural and remote areas. It is an effective alternative to face-to-face treatment, and patients have accepted the technology without feeling estranged (Hilty et al. 2000/2001). As technology improves and as more bandwidth becomes widely available, the use of telepsychiatry will continue to grow, bringing more services to more people.

Virtual reality is becoming a viable treatment modality or adjunct to treatment for certain disorders, especially in cases in which total immersion in an environment is helpful for learning to overcome anxiety. Programs are used to treat patients who are fearful of heights or afraid to travel or who have other anxiety disorders. Virtual reality is generally used in combination with cognitive-behavioral therapy.

Technology has also changed treatment by making psychiatric and medical information more available and accessible to patients. Today, patients are sophisticated consumers and often come to their physicians with printouts of material found on the Web.

■ MEDICAL EDUCATION

Computer technology has had an effect on medical education over the last decade. Students and residents often take to technological instructional methods—clinical simulations, case-based interactive learning, and multimedia educational programs—more readily than faculty. As technology and programs improve, this trend will continue. Virtual reality will be used for immersion into a clinical environment.

■ CERTIFICATION

The American Board of Psychiatry and Neurology has begun using computerized testing for recertification, and it is expected that initial board examinations will be soon be computerized as well. Indeed, it is likely that in the future, you will be able to take professional examinations (of whatever type) whenever you wish and in widely disseminated proctored locations. This is already the case with the United States Medical Licensure Examination. Results can be obtained faster, and feedback can be very specific in terms of individual knowledge and strengths and weaknesses.

■ LIFELONG LEARNING

There is a broad consensus that careers in the information age require lifelong education (Hall 1996). More and more, people are seeing themselves as perpetual students. This has always been true of the medical profession. Continuing medical education (CME), which was always thought to be the domain of conferences, meetings, and seminars, now involves the Internet and computer-based programs. Interactive CME programs are available on compact disc–read-only memory (CD-ROM), and a wide variety of CME programs and courses are offered on the Internet as well.

■ INVISIBLE TECHNOLOGY

Currently, people have a fascination with technology. Computers will become integrated into people's environments and be less visible as a technology. The computer should become invisible, and the information that it provides should be the point of using the computer. When you drive a car or use the telephone, you generally do not think about the machine or the technology; instead, you think about the end result. As computers become part of so many aspects of daily life, people will be less concerned with how the data came to them and will focus on the information itself.

■ SUMMARY

The future will not be without challenges. Issues of privacy and security will continue to be important as physicians protect the integrity of clinical information. With the Internet, the line between work and leisure has blurred more and more in the profession. Individuals already check their electronic mail (e-mail) at work, at home, in restaurants, and on vacation. There is also the phenomenon of information overload, with persons receiving dozens and dozens of e-mail messages every day. People will need to learn how to negotiate these negative aspects of the information age.

The Internet is global, and physicians' professional communities will continue to expand as a result. Clinicians will connect with colleagues in ways that were considered to be science fiction only a few years ago, and the world will become smaller and much more interesting.

■ REFERENCES

Hall P: Cities in Civilization. London, HarperCollins, 1997

Hilty DH, Nesbitt TS, Hales RE, et al: The use of telemedicine by academic psychiatrists for the provision of care in the primary care setting. Medscape Mental Health (serial on-line) March/April 2000. Available at: http://psychiatry.medscape.com/Medscape/psychiatry/journal/2000/v05.n02/mh4474.hilt/mh4474.hilt-01.html. Accessed December 24, 2001

Pastore M: Physicians' Internet use excludes clinical applications (Markets Healthcare Web site). March 8, 2001. Available at: http://cyberatlas.internet.com/markets/healthcare/article/0,,10101_708321,00.html. Accessed December 24, 2001

Valéry P: Selected Writings of Paul Valéry. New York, Norton, 1964

Wölk C: Virtual treatment of obsessive compulsive disorders (OCD) (Abstract 14), in Program and Abstracts of the First International Symposium on the Internet and Psychiatry, Munich, Germany, April 5–6, 2001. Available at http://www.medscape.com/viewarticle/414643

GLOSSARY

For definitions of terms not listed here, check
http://www.whatis.com.

access time amount of time a hard drive takes to locate and transfer information to or from the computer

alphanumeric consisting of both letters and numbers

Alt (alternate) key computer key that when pressed in combination with other keys expands the traditional keyboard and implements commands

applications programs programs such as word processing, database, or accounting programs

ASCII (American Standard Code for Information Interchange) one of the standards for the computer's internal recognition of the letters, numbers, and symbols of the English language; commonly known as plain text

assembly language language consisting of a series of names (called mnemonics) that represent the various combinations of 1s and 0s that instruct the computer

asynchronous transmission data transmission in characters are transmitted at different intervals

auto dial feature in modems enabling them to dial telephone numbers over the telephone system without manual intervention

backup duplicate copy of a file, program, or disk; or act of creating such a duplicate

bandwidth speed at which data are sent over a network or via the Internet; width of a band of electromagnetic frequencies that describe how fast data travel on a transmission path; proportional to the amount of data transmitted over a unit of time and the complexity of the data (for example, complex multimedia files require more bandwidth to download than do simple text files or simple graphics); expressed as bits per second (bps)

baud   measure of speed of digital transmission

beam   send data over an infrared connection between two personal digital assistants

binary digit   0 or 1, reflecting the use of the binary number system (only two digits); used because the computer recognizes two states: on and off

bit   smallest piece of information a computer can understand; has the value of 1 or 0

bit rate   number of bits transmitted per second; expressed as bits per second (bps)

boot up   initialize a computer system by copying an operating system into the internal memory of the computer from a disk or compact disc–read-only memory (CD-ROM)

bps   bits per second

broadband   relating to a fast Internet connection such as DSL, cable, or satellite

buffer   temporary storage area in the computer's memory

byte   grouping of 8 bits; can be represented by two hexadecimal characters or three octal characters

cable modem   device (not a true modem) that allows your cable television provider to provide you with Internet access; enables you to hook up your personal computer to a local cable television line and receive data at up to 1.5 megabits per second (Mbps), similar to the rate achieved with DSL

cache memory   special random access memory (RAM) that a computer microprocessor can access more quickly than regular RAM; the microprocessor searches cache memory first, to possibly avoid the more time-consuming reading of data in larger memory

cathode-ray tube (CRT)   television tube; a CRT monitor is one type of computer monitor

CD   see **compact disc**

CD-R   see **compact disc–recordable**

CD-ROM   see **compact disc–read-only memory**

CD-RW   see **compact disc–rewritable**

central processing unit (CPU)   processor that manipulates and performs arithmetic operations on data in memory; also executes instructions that control the other processors in the system

character   representation, coded in binary digits, of a letter, number, or symbol

characters per second   measure of rate of data transfer, generally estimated from the bit rate and the character length

chat room   Internet site where users with common interests can communicate in real time; generally does not require use of special software, but users need to register with user names and passwords; logging onto a chat room alerts others currently on-line and in the room that you have entered the room; to interact, you type a message in a text box

chip   integrated circuit that looks like a small black plastic box; microprocessor chips and memory chips are examples

client server   describes the way computers relate to each other over the Internet; sends data to a client who makes a service request of the server; describes the interaction between computers across different locations

cluster   smallest unit of space that the operating system will work with in the file allocation table (FAT); made up of one or more sectors

compact disc (CD)   storage medium using laser optics

compact disc–read-only memory (CD-ROM)   compact disc on which information may only be read

compact disc–recordable (CD-R)   compact disc onto which information may be recorded only once

compact disc–rewritable (CD-RW)   compact disc on which data can be erased and onto which new data can be recorded

Control (CTRL) key   computer key that when pressed in combination with other keys expands the traditional keyboard and implements commands

CPU   see **central processing unit**

crash   act of a system halting; usually destroys unsaved data; can be caused by hardware problems, a software bug, or an act of God

CRT   see **cathode-ray tube**

cursor   indicator to show which character or spreadsheet cell is being accessed; can be a flashing line, a solid inverted letter, or some other noticeable indication

cyberspace   virtual electronic realm of interconnected computers and the society that gathers around them; term was coined by science fiction author William Gibson in his 1984 novel *Neuromancer*

data   information that the computer processes or stores

database   collection of organized data that can be recalled by some index key

digital video disc (DVD)   disc commonly used to store movies; holds 4.7 gigabytes (GB) of information on each side (large enough for a 133-minute movie)

digital video disc–recordable (DVD-R)   digital video disc onto which information may be recorded only once

digital video disc–rewritable (DVD-RW)   digital video disc on which data can be erased and onto which new data can be recorded

digitizer tablet   graphics input device for entering drawings or graphics or working on menus

disk   magnetic storage device (e.g., floppy disk or hard disk)

disk drive   hardware component used to read from and write to a disk

documentation   written instructions to tell you how to use software or hardware

domain name   Internet address consisting of a sequence of names or other words, separated by periods; part of the Domain Name System (DNS) hierarchy

DOS (disk operating system)   software program that controls the hardware and software in a computer

DRAM   see **dynamic random access memory**

DSL (digital subscriber line)   type of Internet access; technology for bringing high-bandwidth information to homes and businesses over ordinary copper telephone lines; speed dependent on proximity to the telephone company's central switching office; data received at speeds of up to 6.1 megabits per second (Mbps); in general use, individual connection speeds are from 1.544 Mbps to 512 kilobits per second (Kbps) downstream and about 128 Kbps upstream; can carry both data and voice signals; data part of the line continuously connected

DVD   see **digital video disc**

DVD-R   see **digital video disc–recordable**

DVD-RW   see **digital video disc–rewritable**

dynamic random access memory (DRAM)   most common kind of random access memory (RAM) for personal computers and workstations

EDO RAM (extended data out random access memory)   random access memory (RAM) that reduces the time needed to read from memory; for faster computers, different types of synchronous dynamic RAM (SDRAM) are recommended

e-mail address   domain-based address, used for electronic mail (e-mail), that is the English-language equivalent of a user's Internet Protocol (IP) number; username@somewhere.com is an example; also called Internet address

e-mail discussion group   discussion group involving distribution of electronic mail (e-mail) from a central computer; anyone with a computer with e-mail capabilities can subscribe

emoticon   symbol used to portray a mood in the very flat medium of electronic mail and other text communications; commonly known as smiley; hundreds of emoticons exist (e.g., :-) [I'm smiling; tilt your head 90 degrees to the left to view])

environment   all of the conditions pertaining to the use of a program, such as the commands used and the look of the screen

export   send information in your program to a file on a disk in the format of another program

extranet   extension of a company's private intranet, using the Internet and public telecommunication systems to communicate data

FAQ (frequently asked question)   question posted on a Web site or within a newsgroup, usually regarding a popular topic and accompanied by an answer

FAT   see **file allocation table**

file   block of data stored on a disk under one name

file allocation table (FAT)   record generated by the operating system that keeps track of where a file is located on the disk

File transfer protocol (FTP)   system for transferring files between computers on the Internet; system most commonly used for downloading software, including the latest shareware releases of popular Internet applications such as Mosaic, Netscape, and Eudora

firewall   set of programs and/or hardware that protects a computer or private network from users from other networks; allows communication out but monitors information coming in and blocks unwarranted access

FireWire   high-performance, high-speed serial bus used to connect devices to a personal computer; permits attachment of up to 63 devices with data-transfer speeds of up to 400 megabits per second (Mbps); also called IEEE 1394

floppy disk   portable storage medium

floppy disk drive   device used to read floppy disks

format (noun)   organization and arrangement of the screen, printed page, or printed output

format (a disk) (verb)   write (on the part of the computer) organizational information on a disk to allow the operating system to write and read data; formatting (also known as initializing) erases all data previously on the disk

friendly   easy to use or learn; said of a program or computer

FTP   see **File transfer protocol**

function keys   computer keys programmed to perform special functions within various application programs

Gbps   gigabits per second

gigabyte (GB)   measure of computer data storage capacity; approximately a billion bytes (2^{30} or 1,073,741,824 bytes)

gigahertz (GHz)   unit of alternating current or electromagnetic-wave frequency, equal to one billion hertz; often used to express a microprocessor's clock speed

graphical user interface (GUI)   physical way, involving use of pictures or icons, to interact with a computer

GUI   see **graphical user interface**

hard disk   see **hard drive**

hard drive   device with magnetic media stored on a disk enclosed in a hard case; also called hard disk

hardware   piece of computer equipment or machinery, such as a printer, keyboard, or disk drive

hertz (Hz)   internationally used unit of frequency equal to one cycle per second

high-level language   computer language that uses English-like commands instead of symbols or numbers

homepage   page of information your browser displays when it is started; page from which all of your excursions to the World Wide Web begin

host   see **node**

HTML   see **hypertext markup language**

HTTP (hypertext transfer protocol)   protocol for setting links to "jump" to other documents; foundation of the World Wide Web

hyperlink   embedded hypertext markup language (HTML) code that allows you to progress or "branch" to other pages of information in a nonlinear fashion; also called hypertext link

hypertext link   see **hyperlink**

Hypertext markup language (HTML)   hypertext document–encoding scheme used for resources published on World Wide Web servers; mixture of ASCII text and special reserved character sequences, called tags, that control formatting of the text; subset of the standard generalized markup language (SGML)

IEEE 1394   see **FireWire**

i-LINK   name used by Sony to specify its FireWire connection

iMac   inexpensive version of the Macintosh; *i* stands for Internet

import   transfer information into a system or program from another system or program

initialize   see **format (a disk)**

input/output (I/O) device   device that reads information into the computer (e.g., a keyboard) or gets information out of the computer (e.g., a printer or monitor) or both (e.g., a disk drive or modem)

Integrated Services Digital Network (ISDN)   direct connection to the Internet through a high-speed telephone line (speeds ranging from 64 to 128 kilobits per second [Kbps])

interface   interconnection between hardware, software, and computer users; for example, an operating system is the interface between the computer, the software, and the user

Internet address   see **e-mail address**

Internet Protocol (IP) address   address identifying a computer that participates in an Internet transaction; issued as either a return address or a destination address; commonly written out as "dotted quads," with the decimal values of the 4 bytes (32 bits) separated by periods (e.g., 192.203.41.101); also called Internet Protocol number

Internet Protocol (IP) number   see **Internet Protocol (IP) address**

Internet Relay Chat (IRC)   system that allows interaction (chatting) among users; follows a set of rules used for client/server software

Internet service provider (ISP)   company that contracts with an individual to provide access to the Internet

interrupt request (IRQ)   internal computer switching device used to interrupt hardware and software when there is an event that requires attention, such as arrival of data at the serial port

intranet   private network that is set up within a company; uses traditional Internet protocols and can be made up of many interlinked local area networks and/or a wide area network; users can also connect to the Internet through gateways

IP address   see **Internet Protocol (IP) address**
IP number   see **Internet Protocol (IP) address**
IRC   see **Internet Relay Chat**
IRQ   see **interrupt request**
ISDN   see **Integrated Services Digital Network**
ISP   see **Internet service provider**

joystick   device used to manipulate a cursor; typically used in games

Kbps (kilobits per second)   measurement of the amount of data flowing in a given time on a data transmission medium; otherwise known as bandwidth; higher bandwidths expressed as megabits per second (Mbps) and gigabits per second (Gbps)
kilobit   1,024 bits
kilobyte (KB)   1,024 bytes; reflects the binary number system; 64-KB memory stores 65,536 bytes of information and programs
kilohertz (kHz)   unit of alternating current or electromagnetic-wave frequency equal to 1,000 hertz; also used to describe bandwidth

L1 (level 1) and L2 (level 2)   levels of cache memory in a computer; caches are usually built onto the microprocessor chip itself
LAN   see **local area network**
LCD   see **liquid crystal display**
legacy free   without older peripherals or connections; essentially, without industry standard architecture (ISA) slots or serial ports
Linux   open-source operating system; essentially a modification of Unix
liquid crystal display (LCD)   display type found in notebook computers and thin display panels for desktop computers
local area network   way to connect computers that are generally in the same location

logical drive   portion of a hard disk that is segmented into a separate area and addressed as a different drive letter

lookup table   area of a spreadsheet that is used to store values

Macintosh (Mac)   first personal computer with a graphical user interface; introduced in 1984 by Apple Computer; powered by the PowerPC microprocessor, which was developed jointly by Apple, Motorola, and IBM; uses a different operating system than that used by IBM-compatible personal computers

Mbps   megabits per second

megabyte (MB)   measure of computer processor storage as well as real and virtual memory; 2^{20} or 1,048,576 bytes; commonly thought of as one million bytes; 10-MB disk stores about 5,000 typewritten pages

megahertz (MHz)   unit of alternating current or electromagnetic-wave frequency, equal to one million hertz; often used to express a microprocessor's clock speed

memory   chips that store programs and data in the computer; either read-only memory (ROM) or read/write memory, known as random access memory (RAM)

menu driven   using menus to select different options a program offers

modem   device that allows digital information from the computer to be transmitted over analog systems such as a telephone

monitor   high-quality television set that displays more text and better graphics than a television screen

motherboard   main circuit board where all the peripherals and parts of the computer connect

mouse   popular pointing device that allows you to interact with a computer

MP3 (MPEG Audio Layer-3)   technology for compressing sound; creates files that are approximately one-twelfth the size of the original file, while preserving the original sound quality; MP3 files have the extension .mp3 and are playable on standard computer media players

MPEG (Moving Picture Experts Group) organization that develops standards for digital video and digital audio compression and that operates under the auspices of the International Organization for Standardization (ISO)

MPEG file high-quality video or audio (MP3) file that is a fraction of its original size

MTBF (mean time between failures) average time a piece of hardware will operate before breaking

Netscape popular World Wide Web browser application; one of the first widely used browsers

network interface card (NIC) card used to connect a computer to a network

newsgroup Internet discussion group centered around a particular subject; comments are written to a central Internet site and redistributed through Usenet, a worldwide network of news discussion groups; permits posting of messages to existing newsgroups, responding to previous posts, and creation of new newsgroups

NIC see **network interface card**

node computer that is attached to a network; also called host

OCR see **optical character recognition**

operating system (OS) software program that loads first in a computer and acts as a central control program for all hardware and software

optical character recognition (OCR) software that recognizes scanned characters to be translated into machine text

packet unit of data routed between an origin and a destination on the Internet or any other packet-switching network; transmitted over the Internet in pieces and then reassembled at the destination or receiving computer

parallel interface interface that sends 8 bits at a time and is used by many printers

PC personal computer

PDA   see **personal digital assistant**

personal digital assistant (PDA)   small device used to store contact information, schedules, and other information

petabyte   measure of memory or storage capacity; 2^{50} bytes or approximately 1,000 terabytes

plotter   printer that draws data on a piece of paper using a pen; can draw on paper of various sizes (letter size to a few feet square)

plug and play (PnP)   ability to plug a device into a computer and have the computer recognize the device; developed for Windows; has always been available on Macintosh systems

PnP   see **plug and play**

pointing device   tool used to manipulate a cursor that displays on a computer screen

printer   device that produces a paper copy of the information your computer generates; ink-jet and laser printers are two types of printers

protocol   system of rules and procedures governing communications between two or more devices; required for exchanging data; data format, readiness to receive or send, error detection, and error correction may be defined in protocols

RAM   see **random access memory**

random access memory (RAM)   memory that can be written into and read from; loses contents when power is turned off; stores the user's programs and data while the computer is on

read-only memory (ROM)   memory programmed (read into) once and subsequently only read from; does not lose contents when power is turned off; programmed by the manufacturer; program in ROM also called firmware

ROM   see **read-only memory**

SCSI (Small Computer System Interface)   computer interface standard defining standard physical and electrical connections for devices; allows many kinds of devices (e.g., disk drives, magneto-optical disks, compact disc–read-only memory [CD-ROM] drives, and tape drives) to interface with the host computer

SDRAM   see **synchronous dynamic random access memory**

serial interface   interface that sends one bit at a time; often connects a modem, mouse, or personal digital assistant; legacy interface that is being replaced by universal serial bus (USB)

server   computer that shares its resources, such as printers and files, with other computers on a network

SMS protocol   short messages sent by mobile telephones; set of instructions to send interactive messages via mobile telephones

SRAM   see **static random access memory**

static random access memory (SRAM)   memory that provides faster access to data than dynamic random access memory (DRAM); unlike DRAM, holds data in memory and does not need to be refreshed periodically

streaming video   compressed video transmitted over the Internet and displayed as it arrives; uncompressed at the point of use; streaming media is streaming video with sound; with streaming video or streaming media, no waiting for the entire file to download to see or hear a file

subscribe   add your name to an e-mail discussion group or newsgroup

synchronous dynamic random access memory (SDRAM)   memory synchronized with the clock speed of the microprocessor; increases the number of instructions that the processor can perform in a given time; speed rated in megahertz rather than in nanoseconds

TCP/IP (tranmission control protocol/Internet Protocol)   the two fundamental packet-oriented network communication protocols of the Internet; software stacks available for nearly every kind of central processing unit and operating system; most built into the operating system or available free; other Internet protocols for terminal emulation, file transfer, electronic mail, news, and information publishing are layered on TCP/IP

telnet   Internet standard protocol for remote terminal connection service; allows a user at one site to interact with a remote system as if the user's terminal were directly connected to it

terabyte   measure of computer storage capacity; 2^{40} or approximately 1,000 gigabytes

terminal   device whose keyboard and display are used for sending and receiving data over a communications link; unlike a microcomputer, has few or no internal processing capabilities

throughput   amount of user data transmitted per second

trackball   variant on the mouse; essentially a pointing device

universal serial bus (USB)   serial bus used to connect devices to a personal computer; supports a data speed of 12 megabits per second (Mbps); accommodates a wide range of devices (e.g., a mouse or a scanner); supports plug and play and allows devices to be plugged in and unplugged without rebooting; allows multiple devices to be connected through the same port; new version (USB2) supports data speed of up to 480 Mbps and older USB devices

Unix   operating system typically used on servers, mainframe computers, and workstations

unsubscribe   remove your name from an e-mail discussion group or newsgroup

URL (uniform resource locator)   method for specifying the exact location of an Internet resource (typically a file) and the network protocol necessary to retrieve and interpret the resource; for example, the URL http://www.peds.csmc.edu/readme.html indicates a file named README.HTML residing on an Internet host named www.peds.csmc.edu

USB   see **universal serial bus**

Usenet   virtual collection of thousands of topically named newsgroups, the computers that run the protocols, and the people who read and submit Usenet news; not all Internet hosts subscribe to Usenet, and not all Usenet hosts are on the Internet

VFS   see **virtual file system**

virtual file system (VFS)   system developed for use on Palm operating system devices that allows files to reside beyond the typical central memory core; allows plug-in memory cards and other modules to integrate easily with the Palm operating system

virtual private network (VPN)   private data network that makes use of the public telecommunication infrastructure; privacy is maintained through use of a tunneling protocol and security procedures; connections offer security and allow remote users to access files and data that would normally be blocked by a firewall

VPN   see **virtual private network**

Wais (wide-area information server)   database retrieval system on the Internet that supports full-text searches

WAN   see **wide area network**

Web browser   program that retrieves Hypertext Markup Language (HTML) documents from Web servers using the hypertext transfer protocol (HTTP) and formats them for display; also interprets hyperlinks within the body of an HTML document and uses them to navigate from one HTML document to another on the same or another Web server

Webmaster   owner, curator, or manager of a Web site; generally, the person who puts together the site and controls the content

Web page   document on the World Wide Web, having a unique address and usually containing links to other documents on computers throughout the world; permits the user to do a variety of tasks, from interactive frog dissection to shopping

Web server   computer on a network that runs a program that understands the hypertext transfer protocol (HTTP) protocol and responds to resource requests from Web browsers using that protocol; must run on an Internet host that is addressable with an Internet Protocol (IP) number and found via its corresponding Domain Name System (DNS) host name; runs on computers often referred to informally as Web servers as well, although the computer may be running many other programs at the same time (including other types of server programs)

wide area network (WAN)   network spanning hundreds or thousands of miles

Windows 2000   commercial version of Windows; previously known as Windows NT 5.0; designed to appeal to small businesses and professionals and to the more technical and larger business market

Windows Me   operating system developed by Microsoft specifically for the home user; reportedly a Windows 98 update with performance improvements and greater stability

Windows XP   operating system released in October 2001; offers significant improvement over previous versions of the Microsoft operating system, building on the Windows 2000 kernel, which offered stability and advanced networking; comes in professional and home editions

World Wide Web (WWW)   conceptual construct, rather than a physical entity, invented by physicists at the European Laboratory for Particle Physics; contains corporate, institutional, and personal information; includes all Web servers on the Internet, but there is no central administration or coordination of servers; each server is identified by a Domain Name System (DNS) host name; each document or other resource on a Web server is designated by a uniform resource locator (URL)

WWW   see **World Wide Web**

INDEX

*Page numbers printed in **boldface** type refer to tables or figures.*

154